LET NO ONE FEAR
DEATH

LET NO ONE FEAR DEATH

uncutmountainpress.com

Cover Artwork: Icon of the Resurrection, 15th century, Monastery of Chora, Constantinople.

Scriptural quotations are primarily taken from the King James Version unless otherwise stated. The authors may have emended some quotations to better reflect the original Greek text.

Library of Congress Cataloging-in-Publication Data
Let No One Fear Death—1st ed.
Edited by Webster, Fr. Alexander F. C., PhD and Heers, Fr. Peter D.Th.

ISBN: 978-1-63941-007-1

I. Orthodox Christianity
II. Current Events

"We must truly love to overcome fear and to inspire others to do the same."

—Metropolitan Jonah (Paffhausen)

CONTENTS

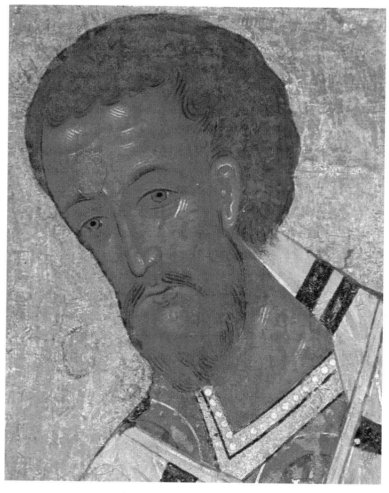

St. John Chrysostom

PUBLISHER'S NOTE

One of the roles of an Orthodox Christian publisher is to provide a platform to faithful and enlightened members of the Church to communicate to their fellows the hope that is within them (1 Peter 3:5). The urgency to meet this need was intensified by the sudden en masse, indiscriminate appropriation and promotion of a message of fear, the fear of death, during the recent "pandemic" of 2020-2022. This state of things thus further amplified the call to fulfill our role, and do our duty to the faithful.

It is, then, an honor and a privilege for Uncut Mountain Press to be the publisher of this aptly-titled volume of essays, Let No One Fear Death, by which the authors aim to encourage and equip their brethren with a right understanding of fear and to what it must be directed — and not directed. The importance of properly discerning matters here cannot be overstated. Missing the mark in this case is no simple error; rather it indicates that one is generally disoriented and eternity is not the aim.

May all the pious readers of these essays gain much strength from on high to enjoy the "fountain of life" which is the fear of the Lord and to thus "depart from the snares of death" (Proverbs 14:27), attaining that "perfect love" which "casteth out fear" (1 John 4:18), that they may chant with the angels, "O fear the LORD, ye his saints: for there is no want to them that fear him" (Psalms 34:9)!

Archpriest Peter Heers
May 14, 2022
Feast of Saint Therapon of Cyprus

PREFACE

The co-editors owe the main title of this book and the idea of the project itself to Protodeacon Patrick Mitchell at St. John the Baptist Russian Orthodox Cathedral in Washington, DC. When he chose to withdraw from the project in August 2021, we decided that this project was too important to die a premature death. After a turbulent half year of other prospective chapter authors bowing out and the recruitment of new contributors, including the generous consent of a renowned Orthodox hierarch to write a chapter, we arrive finally at the present volume.

The final group of contributors is, we are convinced, blessed by our Lord to work together and share our thoughts, insights, questions, suggestions, and judgments concerning the vexing problems that have swirled around the COVID-19 crisis (we hesitate to call it a true "pandemic"), above all the fear of death and panic. The grace, humility, and collegiality of the four other participants—Metropolitan Jonah (Paffhausen), M.Th., Presvytera Katherine Baker, Irene Polidoulis, M.D., and Deacon Ananias Erik Sorem, Ph.D.—each one highly qualified in his or her own field of study or endeavor, has been a joy to behold. We hope that spirit shines forth from each of the chapters in this book.

The six contributors to this project have produced, we hope, an inspirational and useful collection of essays that attempt to address many of the questions and concerns arising from the COVID-19 crisis during the last two years. All of us share a deep and abiding faith in our Lord God and Savior Jesus Christ, a profound love for the Holy Orthodox Church throughout the world and our fellow Orthodox Christians, and a firm commitment to good citizenship and the public interest in the United States of America or Canada.

Our mission is both academic and personal. We hope that the scholarly expertise that we—each of us from our chosen fields of medicine, philosophy, moral theology, or spirituality—offer in this slim volume will contribute to the ongoing discussions of the COVID-19 crisis that have beset our two nations and the world longer than anyone expected. We hope also that the personal experiences and perspectives we share herein will touch souls deeply troubled by the recent course of events and encourage everyone to keep the faith and to stay the course in this fight.

For we know full well that this crisis entails a battle against powerful persons and forces working with all their might to instill in us fear, panic, and submission instead of hope, serenity, and self-determination. We know, too, that we must also confront the spiritual "principalities and powers" behind the earthly variety. We know, most of all, and trust the divine wisdom displayed by St. John Chrysostom in his inimitable Paschal Homily: *"Let no one fear death, for the death of the Savior has set us free."*

Archpriest Alexander F. C. Webster, Ph.D.
Protopresbyter Peter A. Heers, D.Th.
February 10, 2022

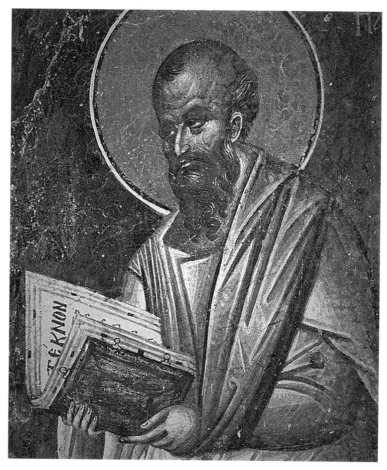

St. Paul the Apostle

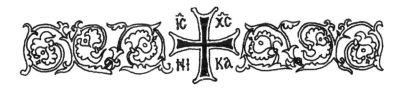

CHAPTER 1

The Orthodox Church and the COVID-19 Crisis

Metropolitan Jonah (Paffhausen)

The past two years have been dominated by the COVID-19 crisis—the pandemic that has afflicted the world and caused immense suffering, death, and demoralization. We fully acknowledge the tragedies and suffering caused by this virus, and how it has reshaped society on a worldwide basis, from the personal and family level, to churches, social and political life, and international relations. We extend our compassion to those who have lost loved ones, to those who have suffered from the virus or co-suffered to care for them, to those who have lost their livelihoods, and to many who have lost hope.

The Church has also suffered through these trials with the deaths of many clergy, elders, monastics, and lay members, and with the many who became ill from the virus. The senior clergy of the Orthodox Church in Russia were particularly hard hit, as were those in other Orthodox Churches. A spirit of fear gripped large parts of the population, both those in authority as well as the lay people. Churches were closed, Liturgy was cancelled or prohibited to many, mask mandates were imposed, and even vaccination cards were required as a criterion for admittance. Priests were threatened for non-compliance, churches were threatened by the secular authorities, and people began to lose faith as they lost hope.

It is not so much that people lost faith in Christ. They lost faith in the Church—in the bishops and clergy—and in the stability that the uninterrupted celebration of the Eucharist conveyed to their lives. For many people, the church was their only social outlet, but, suddenly, it was cut off. Liturgy was turned into a YouTube video. Even the live streaming of the Liturgy became a means of surveillance, so the bishop could see who was conforming to the COVID-19 restrictions and who was not. Bishops were terrified that churches might become centers for the spread of the disease and acted as they thought best. Clergy were horrified that they might be prohibited from serving the Liturgy, and that their churches would be either completely closed or accessible by only a few. Sometimes the clergy rebelled, permitting the faithful to venerate icons or worship without a mask, but lived in fear of retribution from their bishop, such as suspension or defrocking. In some places the authorities threatened not only to close the churches for non-compliance, but even to shut off utilities and confiscate church property. Everyone lived in fear. This fear broke down the network of personal relations that held the parish church together.

Not only the faithful, but the entire populations of the United States and Canada, were afflicted with fear. The very network that holds together the community of churches, towns, cities, states, and countries, began to crumble as people lost faith in their leaders, not knowing who or what to believe, or if anyone could be trusted to tell the truth.

The churches on the basic level, and society itself on multiple levels, require a foundation of trust and faith. This means both faith in the integrity of the leadership and trust in the content of what they are not only saying, but how leaders have reached their conclusions. Part of that trust is based on the sense that the leaders genuinely care for the people and will not betray them, especially to profit from them. The other part of that trust is based on faith in the trustworthiness of the leaders' information.

The COVID-19 crisis unfolded at the same time as the United States was experiencing a period of profound political polarization during its 2020 elections. The political platforms were diametrically opposed in many areas, particularly on ethical issues. Neither side trusted the integrity of the other, setting the stage for a political polarization that extended well beyond those elections. This led to mistrust between those who held opposing points of view in every sector of society, regarding everyone in authority from presidential candidates and governors to bishops and priests within the church. Could their decisions be trusted?

This crisis of confidence came together in 2021 around the issue of the novel COVID-19 vaccines and their medical, moral, religious, spiritual, political, economic, and other social and organizational dimensions. Medically, the mRNA vaccines are new, and it will be several years before they can be tested by time to ensure they do not have late or long-lasting side effects. Many people are claiming to have been harmed or to have lost a loved one because of these vaccines. Many unvaccinated died but many more survived, while many who got vaccinated still contracted COVID-19. These concerns raise questions for which we do not yet have genuine answers.

What did our political and religious leaders believe about the virus itself, the subsequent lockdowns, the masks, the vaccines, or the mandates? In every sector, the political polarization created a crisis of faith and trust in political and Church leadership at all levels. The Orthodox faithful began to lose hope as they lost faith in government and other institutions. They lost trust in the ever changing "science" that purported experts promulgated and in official decisions by political and Church leaders that shattered their lives.

While the vaccine itself is a major issue on many levels, the other dimensions of this crisis are also of great import. For example, governments claim the right to demand vaccination, which for many, is a major issue of civil and constitutional rights and freedoms. Many have deep political and / or religious convictions concerning personal freedoms and sovereignty over their own physical heath. Despite those convictions, many Americans and Canadians have suffered adverse consequences for not submitting to the government mandates, including loss of one's job and livelihood, or being segregated and excluded from entering public schools, restaurants, gyms, and other public places—in other words, prohibited from earning a living or living a normal life. The COVID-19 crisis and its mandates have excluded people from churches, from family gatherings, and from social events. For tens of thousands, it is not just the loss of a job but the loss of a lifelong career that has been at stake. Thousands of American patriots with many years of honorable service in the U.S. armed forces have suffered military discharges or the threat of separation, because they resisted the mandates or the vaccines for religious, ethical, or personal health reasons. While many have lost jobs and careers, others have become very wealthy because of this pandemic. The fear of death from the virus has metastasized into fear of losing one's position in life itself.

We confront a profound crisis of faith. Many of those who believe government officials and the mass media and have capitulated to their mandates are also pushing the hardest for retribution against those who resist. Those who do *not* believe the politicians, the media, or the technocrats reject both the vaccine and the mandates that violate their fundamental rights. They have no faith in those who would force the vaccine on those who do not desire it. It is a matter of moral conscience, of personal choice, based on the deep religious conviction not to accept any medical vaccine that has utilized in its development, production, or testing phases, fetal cell lines derived from aborted preborn babies. For the same religious and moral reasons, faithful Christians understandably reject and deplore any exploitation of aborted preborn babies for scientific and medical research and their organs and cell lines for the development of any medicines or other products.

As we strive to overcome and survive this pandemic crisis, we continue our journey through a "brave new world." Fear of the coronavirus and COVID-19 disease has perpetuated this crisis. The fear of death and panic have led many millions of otherwise decent, rational people to despair. But, as Christians, we have no need to despair

How do we put our world back together?

Whom do we believe?

What do we believe is true?

In this collection of essays, respected Orthodox Christians, both clergy and laity, examine the COVID-19 crisis from multiple disciplines and Orthodox perspectives: spiritual, moral, philosophical, medical, and personal. As we read these essays, it is important to consider how the pandemic and the authors' responses to its various aspects have been shaped.

Some will ignore their messages, while others will take them into account. Either way, we must all deal with the adverse results: churches that have lost significant membership, a breakdown in trust for the hierarchy and other institutions; and an erosion of confidence in governing bodies.

As Orthodox Christians, the authors of the chapters in this book and readers alike know how to trust the Orthodox Faith as given to us by Christ and the Holy Fathers and conveyed to us by those who manifest the authentic transformation in Christ that is sanctity and deification. We truly desire to follow the pronouncements of the Church and to believe our bishops and priests, for whom we pray each week during Divine Liturgy.

For all Orthodox Christians, the centrality of our Faith is that Jesus Christ has truly risen from the dead and has overcome death. We no longer have reason to fear death because Christ has overcome it. Yes, the body dies. But we remain alive in Christ, and the body will be resurrected to eternal life. As the New Testament reveals, "*through fear of death we were subjected to life-long slavery*" (Hebrews 2:15)[1]. The COVID-19 crisis is precisely an example of that. We are subjected to slavery by fear of death through a spreadable disease. It is through fear that many submit to slavery, tyranny, false ideals (technocracy) and false religions (scientism). But there is no reason to fear!

Do we Christians not believe in Jesus Christ and His Resurrection?

As St Paul tells us in Romans 14:7-9, "*None of us lives to himself, and none of us dies to himself. For if we live, we live to the Lord, and if we die, we die to the Lord; so then, whether we live or*

---

1. Scriptures in this chapter taken from the English Standard Version.

whether we die, we are the Lord's. For to this end Christ died and lived again, that he might be Lord both of the dead and of the living."

Our Lord Jesus Christ Himself declares, *"I am the resurrection and the life. Whoever believes in me, though he die, yet shall he live, and everyone who lives and believes in me hall never die. Do you believe this?"* (John 11:25)

We shall not find the answers to the questions of this crisis of faith and trust in our political, social, or academic structures, our secular leaders, or even in one another. Those answers will not even come from the hierarchy or the structures of the Church, except if there is true repentance on their part. It is only through courageous faith in Jesus Christ, by putting aside our fear of death and suffering, and by acting with integrity that we may begin the process of reconciliation and the rebuilding of our faith and our trust.

This requires humility. It demands repentance. It means stepping out in love to bring us all together to work out again how to live and cooperate with one another.

In his first epistle the Apostle John assures us: *"Perfect love casts out fear."* (1 John 4:18). We must truly love to overcome fear and to inspire others to do the same.

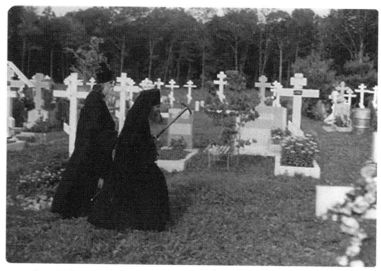

St. John Maximovich going through cemetery

CHAPTER 2

A Pandemic Observed

Presvytera Katherine Baker

We buried my baby in a wooden box in the crook of the arm of his father. My husband was thirty-seven and had died in a car accident coming home from his work as an Orthodox priest in a sudden snowstorm on a Sunday afternoon in March. My son was born at twenty weeks gestation, about two weeks before his father's death, but the ground was too frozen to bury him in the cemetery plot just then, so the funeral home offered to keep the tiny body until spring. But when his father died too, the funeral director et al. decided it was worth the use of the special machines used to thaw the ground for a winter burial in New England; and so there was some comfort in knowing the two would lie together.

My husband's face had been destroyed in the accident which took him on the Feast of Holy Orthodoxy, the day we celebrate the restoration of the icons to the use of the church after the iconoclast heresy had attempted to remove all images from worship. My ten-year-old son had recently painted an icon of the Holy Face of Christ which he decided to place in the coffin with his father thinking it would suffice to provide a face for his dad. It was good theology for a ten-year-old, the second-born of his theologian father, as it is in

Christ that any of us can hope to have any wholeness at all. The strange coincidence of the feast on which my husband died often strikes me as painfully ironic but on my best days, it is a hopeful sign of the restoration of those faces, someday, in the Resurrection.

Though the car skidded on the ice and rolled three times, coming to rest in on-coming traffic, in a strange miracle, my six children, who were with my husband at the time, not only survived but were completely unharmed except for one black eye and one scratched finger needing only a small band-aid. The emergency personnel on site tended to my children immediately, but my husband was killed instantly because he was thrown from the vehicle. At the time, I was at home recovering from the miscarriage.

While planning for his funeral, I learned that priests are buried with their faces covered by the *aer*, which is the cloth that covers the gifts of bread and wine offered during the Divine Liturgy. This is to signify the shroud of Christ and the offering of the priest back to God as a sacrifice. A regular open casket could take place, as usual, with his face covered. His hands with the freckles and the fuzz of reddish hair were the only visual aspects left to assure me it really was him — that, and the strange way his shoes turned out in that duck way they always did from a hip abnormality he had from birth. It added a strange comedy to the solemn scene of his church funeral.

And so he was buried, and a carved stone icon of the Resurrection was placed over his head, and we all marveled that God had decided to take so remarkable a person: son and brother, husband, father of six living children, dear friend to many, a musician, and a poet, soon to get his PhD in theology, and recently recognized for his intellectual work by some of the leading minds of his field, he was recently ordained and assigned to his first parish only six weeks prior. As a priest from our former parish said, "as we have buried such a dear seed, from it we expect a tremendous harvest."

Three of my children and myself encountered our first known COVID-19 case on the five-year anniversary of my husband's death but did not hear about the exposure for over a week. I looked to my six children and wondered if any or all of them would be the next to lie with their Daddy and brother, or if I would be the one to leave them totally orphaned. Now that the oldest was seventeen and the youngest seven, we had finally settled into daily regularity, though I still struggled daily with a deep darkness.

As I watched the pandemic and lockdown play out, I observed it from a place of intimacy with death and mourning. Very often I wondered if that was the case for our leaders and decision makers. It appeared to me that death was being approached officially as an anomaly instead of a certainty, and disease was treated like a strange exception instead of the rule. We ticked off each COVID-19 death one by one through mass media in a way never done with any other cause of death before.

Of course, this seemed justified at the time, because, in a pandemic, each death is another piece of the puzzle. It helps us to understand the disease. To be fair, in the early days, we had no idea what the disease might do. But I began to worry about our nation's response to the disease, when our own self-imposed family quarantine was over. The lockdowns were in full swing, and people in authority allowed no discussion of exit strategies without accusations that anyone considering reopening to a more normal sort of life simply did not care about humanity.

It seemed that so many were willing to make a bargain with whoever might be offering, that they would do anything to save others from sickness and death. While this was certainly generous and completely understandable (and I am sure I, too, would have been tempted by it before I had lost my husband and child), it caused me alarm now that I was already in mourning. I could see that these well-meaning, deeply loving people simply could not imagine life without their dear ones and so they were ready to make *any* sacrifices asked of them to keep death at bay.

I totally identified with the contradictory and confused feelings of the bereaved C.S. Lewis, in *A Grief Observed* when he said about the loss of his wife, "her absence is like the sky spread over everything" but elsewhere saying the loss is, "like an amputation." Both are true. But as a mourning person it is my personal daily struggle to go on living the best I can, with myself and my world utterly altered.

In our fear of death, we simply do not want to think about what happens after our loved ones die, but we must. We seem to be willing, in our understandable terror, to trade away many essential things: basic freedoms, our public life and public institutions for the promise of greater safety from sickness and death, but when that sickness and death come anyway (as it must), what will we do when we find we have made the world worse than it otherwise might have been? If we trade the beauty and order of our society for *safety*, not only will we find we have lost our dear ones anyway, but we will also sit and mourn them in a desolate land of our own making.

There is a dark part of us all that wants the world to match the pain we feel. This is the primary work of mourning people: to refuse bitterness, to choose life every moment we can (and repent when we fail) and refuse to make the entire world worse just because we are hurting. The world is already a graveyard; it does not have to be hell.

The real tragedy is not a person dying young, but a person whose life becomes a kind of death. Those people are truly, "dead before their time." My husband was not dead before his time. He had really lived right up to the last moment and accomplished so much.

In the intervening five years, I have, at times, upbraided myself for all the ways I could have kept my baby and my husband alive. I concoct alternative scenarios in which we would all be at home before the snow started falling and I would have taken better care of myself to keep from having a miscarriage; but I know this is a dangerous line of reasoning. While surely some of my choices and my husband's choices did indeed affect the result, to place all the blame for accidental death on a survivor just results in that person too, succumbing to a torturous depression that is a kind of death in life.

Just as it is counterproductive to suggest to a woman who has miscarried that she continue to ruminate on all the ways she might have been responsible for her child's death, or suggest to a spouse or caregiver that they might have done something different to save their loved one, it is also wrong to suggest to everyone that they should tear themselves up with guilt over the deaths of the most fragile. "Are not two sparrows sold for a copper coin? And not one of them falls to the ground apart from your Father's will . . . . So do not be afraid; you are worth more than many sparrows" (Matthew 10:30).

The pandemic has demanded that we siphon all our lives through the internet. The corporal works of mercy seem to have become incorporeal, better to be filtered through Big Tech. Someone is making a lot of money when we funnel all our relationships, commerce, education, recreation and even worship through a third party. This new disembodied way of living is an effort to be "safe," but Christ's example suggests we must become more embodied, not less. We already know that however safe living on the internet might make us from some kinds of physical threats, the new cancel culture and persistent internet aggression has opened whole new ways to devastate and be devastated.

Avoiding the pain of my own life, I find the lure of being dis-incarnated very seductive. The internet — that glittering indulgence of the eyes — is an infinite stream of the finite, wherein you can pretend to lose your loss, and your body with its limitations. There, I can temporarily avoid some of the pain of my present life.

However, God Himself, pure spirit, became a real man with a real body. It is a continuing argument I have with Him that He took the bodies of my dear love and child from me, while He insists on the Incarnation of Himself. My argument with God goes something like this: You say it is so important to be incarnated, to become a human with a body and yet you expect me to be satisfied with this husband and son of mine whose living bodies are gone from me? You expect me to commune with them as far away spirits while you lived as a man. Which is it, God? Is it good to be incarnated or not? To which I wonder if God's response to my objections might be this: *"Your dissatisfaction, my dear, is exactly My point. This is not the end. We await the Resurrection of the body."*

St. Paul says that Christ died and rose again to set us free from our fear of death, which is a kind of slavery that has held us in bondage from the beginning (Hebrews 2:15). How do we understand the lives of the martyrs in a pandemic? *"They endured mocking and flogging, chains and imprisonment. They were stoned, sawn in two, put to death by sword. They went around... destitute, oppressed and mistreated,"* says St Paul. But he concludes, *"The world was not worthy of them"* (Hebrews 11:37).

Pandemics were quite common throughout history and, through those times, the saints went right on fulfilling Christ's commands to feed and clothe, care for, and love others. It is very possible some disease was spread through the charitable acts of the saints if it was God's will. It is not that those saints were too uneducated to know that this could happen; it is that they made a conscious choice to care for others in a physical way despite the risks to themselves and even the risks to those they cared for. Why did they do this? Because the people around them who asked for their embodied love needed that embodied love more than they needed long lives free of suffering.

Even though humans make choices that are real, no sickness or death happens without God's permission or involvement... or at least Christians used to believe this. Forcible, physical segregation and perpetual isolation is the customary punishment. Are we so sure that the negative outcomes of these safety measures will not outweigh the positive?

Tertullian of Carthage wrote in the late second century, "The blood of the martyrs is the seed of the church." Christians are widely known as those people who did not practice abortion, euthanasia, or suicide. They considered life precious, but their saints famously did not pursue the lengthening of their own individual lives to the detriment of their own souls, nor the souls of others. The martyrs did not count their own physical deaths as much compared to what awaited them (Romans 8:18); and that is not because they undervalued this present life. Christian saints often laid down their lives for other people but there were also some things they simply would not do—like worship idols—not even to save a life, not even the life of their own child. If we want to be people of integrity, we must imitate their example.

I fully expect, if we are living as Church, there could be large outbreaks of COVID-19 in Christian communities as in any other human encounter, should God will it. Dietrich Bonhoeffer said, "When Christ calls a man, He bids him come and die." And if the authorities blame us as "super-spreaders," it would not be the first time in history.

No one blames a person for going to the store for groceries and spreading or picking up germs there, but religious worship since the advent of the COVID-19 crisis often seems more like a concert online than the "daily bread" to which our Savior refers in the Lord's Prayer. Gathering for Sunday liturgy and fellowship in person should be a help to facing the possibility of death, which is exactly what we need right now. A priest's job is not to keep me alive; it is to help me live and die well.

Christians should never judge someone who chooses safety from suffering and death, as did the early Donatist heretics who cast out of the church those who fled persecution. However, Christians should neither judge nor exclude those who choose honorable risk either. A principle of non-judgment is our example. We should reject force and manipulation whether that force or manipulation is in favor of risk or against it.

My husband wrote in a sermon shortly before his death: "God created man in the year 33, on a hill called Golgotha." Christ declared his mighty work "accomplished" from the agony of the cross. It is in union with Christ that we become who we ought to be, and so how can we escape death when even Christ did not? In one of his last sermons, my husband suggested to his flock, "[M]ay we make our own these words of St. Ignatius of Antioch, written to his fellow Christians on his way towards martyrdom for refusing the idolatry of pagan Rome: '*It is better for me to die in Christ Jesus than to be king over the ends of the earth . . . The pains of birth are upon me. Allow me, my brethren; hinder me not from living, do not wish me to be stillborn . . . Allow me to imitate the passion of my God . . . when I shall have arrived there, I shall become a human being.*'" (Epist. ad Rom., 6).

The week my husband died, I heard one of my younger children ask my oldest, who was twelve years old at the time and had been sitting in the front seat during the accident, why he didn't *tell Daddy to put on his seatbelt because that would have saved his life*! Alarmed, I immediately told the children that we were not to ask such questions. God decides when people die. Daddy usually wore his seatbelt. It is a mystery to me why he did not put it on that day. I see before me an entire nation of people being encouraged to ask similar terrible questions of themselves and others. There is a great mystery between God's will and human freedom. We should not pretend to understand something we do not. Christians have never held that death is only a game of chance. It is unconscionable to burden people with guilt for the deaths of others just for going about their lives, especially for the deaths of the most fragile, when death awaits us all.

The night before the accident I found that the middle bench seat in our van was not properly latched into the floor. I tried many times to get the seat to engage into the floor, but it would not budge. The seats were stuck in an unlocked position, the red plastic warning showing. As my fingers became numb with cold, I finally said a prayer, "God protect my children," and I did the sign of the cross. When I went to the wrecked van after the accident, the seat was locked into the floor as it should be: the red plastic warning no longer showed on the dashboard. At some point before the rollover, it had locked itself into place and the children were uninjured.

I must believe that the death of my husband and my unborn son were the will of God. To do otherwise would not only cause me to degenerate into someone I do not wish to become, but it would also be a denial of my faith. I could choose to take total responsibility for those deaths, but practically speaking what would that accomplish for my children other than my own disintegration? I could blame my husband for his own death or for endangering our children, but how would that help? I know he loved them and me deeply and I know he valued his own life. Any mistakes he might have made that contributed to his own death he certainly paid for, crushed against that hard surface of reality.

I could blame someone else for his death or my child's death: family members, friends, doctors, highway workers, but that would only multiply the destruction. God alone knows the level of anyone's culpability in their own deaths and the deaths of others. Even when we know that someone has contributed to a death or perpetrated a murder directly, Christians teach that God is ready to forgive. When it comes to causes of death, we must refrain from judgment and throw ourselves upon the mercy of God, or risk making the already bereaved as dead as the people they miss.

God gave human beings freedom with which they often create chaos, hatred, and torture, but it is by that same power of freedom that we also love. God took an extraordinary risk in His great benevolence. Human freedom has created no end of misery, and it is easy to blame God for the evil that humans create with their freedom. Is it God's fault if we continually use for evil the tools He gave us for good?

God not only risked the loss of our souls to give us the capacity to love, but He also took that risk even further in the Incarnation, wherein His pure spirit took on flesh that died, just as ours will. We cannot avoid death, but we do have a choice about how we should spend our life. Should we squander it, buried like the gold from the Parable of the Talents (Matthew 25), or should we face the risk and live out the adventure of our own lives?

I do not believe, and I think it injurious to me and my children, to behave as if we must avoid the death of the body at *all* costs. Nor do I believe that death is only something that happens if one does not take the proper precautions. Nor do I find it edifying to imagine that the primary way death comes to us is through the normal breathing and natural movement of other people around us. *Even if this is true*, acting it out will inevitably create fear, distrust, segregation, and xenophobia. When we encourage this attitude, we further enslave people to their own inborn fear of death and isolate them from each other.

We never admire the character in a story who will do or say anything to stay alive a little longer, or who pressures other people to put themselves at risk or even die for him or her. We admire the person who, if the normal living and breathing of others could cause him to suffer or even die, would rather risk suffering and death than ask someone else to stop living and breathing for his sake. Of course, this takes a courage we do not actually have—we need grace. A Christian imitates Christ and does not shrink from a fully incarnate life. I fail at this every day. I am terrified of death. But on my better days I am even more afraid of what I could become if I let the fear of death become my master.

In an internet news report on my husband's accident someone wrote in the comments section, "Well, God was not *his* co-pilot! LOL!" While that thoughtless joke represents my own worst temptation, on my better days I believe that the God who can fasten seats to the floor of a vehicle before an accident can also send his angels to remind the driver to put his seatbelt on. Who am I to say God was not with my husband at the moment of his death? I know he prayed for that every day, and I trust God to be merciful.

The question is not *"Will I die?"* or *"Will the people I love die?"* The answer to that has always been "Yes." A better question might be this: *"Will I let the anticipation of death make me and my world, better or worse?"*

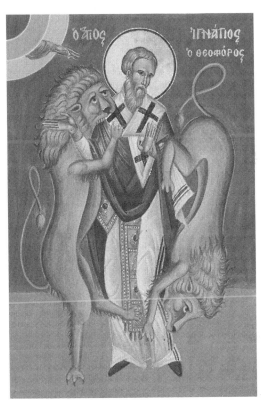

"It is better for me to die in Christ Jesus than to be king over the ends of the earth . . ."
— St. Ignatios of Antioch

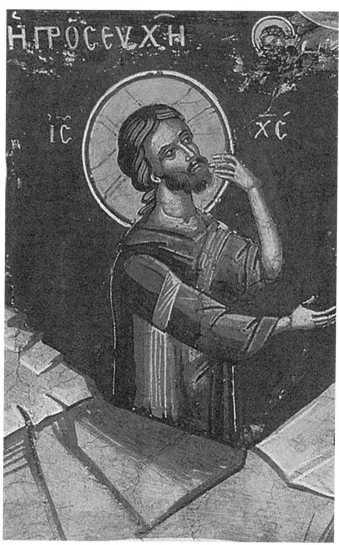

Icon of Christ's agony, praying in the Garden

CHAPTER 3

To Prevent Death, Please Stop Living: An Orthodox Physician Reflects on Death, Fear and the Public Health Measures During COVID-19

Irene Polidoulis, MD, CCFP, FCFP

My parents, ages 89 and 90, stood together on the front porch like perplexed children, their quiet bewilderment in sharp contrast to my vociferous, animated rebukes for doing their own grocery shopping during a pandemic, rather than relying on me. As we stood there two meters apart, my mother, whose cognitive decline had become a little worse of late, surprised me with a teaching moment.

"But what's the difference if I die now or later?" she asked innocently.

I looked at her in astonishment. My medical training had taught me to provide patient centered care, and I, in turn, taught this to my medical learners. My thirty-plus years of experience with the elderly confirmed repeatedly that, in their twilight years, most of them value and choose quality of life over a longer life—hands down. If they must jump through inconvenient, uncomfortable, or time-consuming hoops to extend their time here on earth, they would much rather experience no hoops at all followed by a speedier death. The older they get, the less willing they are to stop living life to the fullest, even if it means dying sooner. Ironically, this is exactly what the public health measures have been asking us all to do, especially in support of the elderly.

Only if I tell my elderly patients that the intervention can maintain or *improve* their quality of life and not simply *prolong* it, only *then* are they willing to listen to an explanation of what that intervention entails. This should not be surprising to a physician who is familiar with palliative care, for these same principles also apply there. At the end of life, most patients prefer a more comfortable and earlier demise to a difficult and drawn-out dying process, just to stay alive a little longer. Their loving families also want the same and there are very few exceptions.

It should have come as no surprise to me, then, that my mother (and father) was no different. They knew they were very blessed to be living independently even in their early nineties, in their bungalow of fifty-two years, and they valued keeping it that way for as long as possible. Giving up independent grocery shopping meant giving up freedom. To them, a pandemic was no worse (in fact, it was much better) than WWII fighter planes dropping bombs in the city where they both grew up. Life still went on, and as well as it could, so did living.

"But," I continued, "what if you get very sick and end up in the hospital? We will not be able to visit you. You will be all alone, and if you died, you would die *alone*."

"Everyone dies alone," my mother chuckled, as though it were common knowledge. "No one shares their death with anyone else."

I was taken aback again because deep down, I also knew this to be true. Sharing death is not like sharing a bad tasting sandwich that you can just cut in half and only experience half the misery of eating it. When I reflect on mass murders, mass executions, mass deaths in wars or accidents, isn't everyone's dying experience his or her own? When the atomic bombs dropped on Hiroshima and Nagasaki, most of the estimated 210,000 fatalities occurred instantly, but they all died individually, on their own, alone, even if they were in a crowd. Isn't that what it means to be *alone in a crowd?*

When I was learning to swim in my middle age, my daughter helped me overcome my fear of jumping into the deep end of the pool by doing it with me. We held hands and jumped. We shared the jump. One could say the experience was the same. It may have looked the same, but it was not. I was frightened and she was not. It was my first time, but not hers. After the jump, our hands separated in the water so that we could both resurface. We came back up individually, having experienced the same physics and the same water at the same place and time, but with entirely different expectations, different emotions, different reactions, and different thoughts. We did the same thing together, but we did not have the same experience, nor did we have half the experience.

Every death is different as well, both for the departing and those left behind, and some deaths are harder than others.

In my experience, the dying often report visions of their parents, or other loved ones who have died before them, looking happy or radiant. Sometimes the visions are heavenly and sometimes demonic. Relatives often tell me their dying loved one stares into the distance, seemingly oblivious to what may be happening around them. Secular medicine calls these experiences *hallucinations*. Orthodox Christians believe they are a foretaste of the destination of the soul. It is the demonic visions that I find troubling, and the dying process tends to be harder when this is the case. If the family is religious, I recommend a visit from a spiritual care provider. If they are Orthodox Christians, I encourage Holy Confession and Communion with a priest. I do this regardless, but especially when there are unpleasant experiences during the dying process.

I have also witnessed other types of difficult or uneasy deaths—people "hanging on to their last breath" as it were—until their loved ones could finally reassure them with words like, "It's OK, we will be fine, you can go now," and immediately they go. Were they hanging on because they feared their death would cause their loved ones too much pain? I believe so: as soon as the loved ones speak those reassuring words, the death is almost instantaneous.

This was not the case, however, with one Orthodox gentleman whose wife and family had already spoken those reassuring words. He was palliatively hospitalized, at the end of his life. Although all his medical test results indicated he should have died days ago, his soul struggled to depart. When I suggested Holy Communion, I discovered that the dying man had not confessed or communed in decades because of his transplant. His anti-rejection drugs chronically compromised his immune system, and he was afraid of catching an infection from the Holy Communion spoon. Over the years, his wife, who had grown accustomed to this, had forgotten about it. She found herself so caught up in her husband's medical struggles that she did not even think about calling a priest. As soon as he received Holy Communion, he relaxed and breathed his last. His soul could not depart without it. I was not there to witness it, but his grateful wife could not stop talking about it. For me this is just one more example of the great love and mercy of our Saviour, who does everything He can without interfering with our freedom. He gifts us with every opportunity, even in our last moments, to bring us Home to Him.

It is debatable whether the dying individual who is unresponsive is aware of the presence of others or can hear or understand what is said. In the movies, we usually see death in a war, a crime, or an accident; the dying person on the screen, who was full of life and vigor moments before, is still able to communicate until his or her last breath. However, most people die of disease or illness. In these instances, death is either very sudden, as in a cardiac arrest, and the dying individual has little opportunity for any form of expression, or death is prolonged, as in a death due to cancer. In the latter instance, the one dying is still unable to respond towards the very end, creating, in effect, a type of "aloneness," even if that person is surrounded by others.

Even in this state of unresponsive "aloneness," some people still seem to prefer dying alone. Countless times I have provided grief counseling to those who lost a family member, because, despite their best efforts, they were not at the bedside at the precise time of death. People feel so guilty over that bathroom break, that drink of water, that snack, that phone call or that nap they so desperately needed, only to return moments later, having just missed the death of their loved one. Despite the countless hours of exhausting vigilance, "I was not there," they mourn.

This has occurred so often in my palliative care experience that, when death is near, I now counsel family members to *expect* their loved one to die when they are not around. For some reason, the dying often seem to prefer it that way, perhaps to avoid experiencing any drama during their departure or to make it easier on their loved ones. I have often heard the older generation commenting on how important it is to *not* make a fuss at the bedside of the dying, because this makes it difficult for the soul to depart peacefully. "It's not good for the soul," they would say, for us "to wail beside the dying person."

In this day and age there is much wailing over COVID-19 deaths, much more so than any other cause of death. Despite all the collateral damage, this pandemic has taken center stage. Deaths due to increased suicide, deaths due to increased drug overdoses, and deaths due to all other diseases, whose treatments have been postponed or even cancelled to prevent the spread of COVID-19, are no less tragic, but they are not talked about as much as COVID-19 deaths. It is quite challenging to find reliable data on the number of deaths due to this disease versus the number of excess non-COVID-19 deaths during this crisis. If the excess non-COVID-19 deaths exceed the deaths due to this disease, then clearly, we, as a society, have done something very wrong, because, in the big picture, we have not prevented any deaths. We have merely replaced some deaths with others and possibly even increased the total death toll by over-focusing on COVID-19, keeping in mind that death (mortality) is *not the only* type of collateral damage. We also need to consider excess non-COVID-19 morbidity (illness) such as the increase in eating disorders and other mental health problems, delayed treatment of illness in general, increased addictions, domestic violence, crime, poverty, etc. Any excess in mortality (death) or morbidity (illness) that societies may have experienced while frantically trying to contain COVID-19 could be the result of a prevailing panic. The Oxford Dictionary defines panic as "*a sudden uncontrollable fear or anxiety, often causing wildly unthinking behaviour.*"

I first saw this type of panic face to face in the workplace during the Sars-Cov-1 outbreak in 2003, since the Scarborough Hospital, the epicentre of that outbreaks was right next door to our clinic. I saw it face to face again in 2020 during a heart-to-heart with my mother-in-law, another family member pushing ninety, but one who is widowed and lives alone. This panic, however, was not hers. My husband and I often tried to convince her to break her isolation by visiting us, but she refused, even for Christmas. Unlike my parents who applied many "grains of salt" to the COVID-19 restrictions in favour of living, my mother-in-law embraced them in excess to prevent her death. This was not for her own sake, but for the sake of her daughter, who had already lost one parent, and who had expressed great fear over her mother dying, and especially dying *alone*. As a result, my mother-in-law accepted groceries delivered to her door, held masked conversations two meters apart over the threshold, and never left her apartment for months on end, not even to attend church service – her favourite activity – even after these were again permitted. The result for her was no exodus from her apartment and no human physical contact for about a year.

She over-complied to diminish someone else's fear. Although she believed her daughter's fears and prohibitions were excessive, she did not wish to upset her children, who she imagined would experience her death in a more agonizing way if she died alone and away from them. The thought of this made her cry. So, she put on a brave face and pretended her prolonged isolation was not that bad. She willfully made a tremendous sacrifice, but her already fragile health deteriorated, edging her closer to that which none of us desired. She lost appetite, weight, and strength, while her increasing depression morphed into chronic pain. Despite her daughter's best intentions, an excessive imposition of the public "health" measures augmented her mother's suffering and frailty, ironically edging them both closer towards that which they each feared the most—a lonely mother dying alone.

This is a classic example of the living worrying about the dying and vice versa. Each tries to protect the other from experiencing any form of pain, but when communication breaks down because of fear, more pain results, often followed by guilt. This crucial point is also part of palliative care counseling, and I am thankful that my sister-in-law realized what was happening to her mother and softened her approach.

During the first wave of COVID-19, my youngest child, in her early twenties, developed a fear of being sick and therefore alone, because of the tragedy that befell our nursing homes. This recalled those times my children would get sick when they were young. As all sick children do, mine clung to me like glue, freely sharing whatever oozed from their eyes, mouths, or noses. The universal mom, myself included, embraces her sick child, stroking, hugging, and kissing the ooze, fully aware that, in a few days, when her child would be back to normal and jumping on the furniture, she would be nursing the flu in bed. This is the naturally human, maternal response.

"My darling," I said to my daughter, without even thinking, "if you ended up in ICU with COVID-19, I would put on my lab coat and my badge and walk right in there and climb into the bed with you. They would not be able to get rid of me because of my exposure to you, and we would quarantine together in ICU." I had no idea how the ICU staff would really react, but it did not matter.

"You'd do that mommy?" she brightened.

"Of course, I would, baby."

And that was the end of it. She believed me because I had done precisely that (except for the ICU and climbing-into-bed parts), when my sister was in labour in 2003 during SARS-Cov-1. I marched in, covered in PPE from head to toe, and sat with her during my lunch break. There are advantages to being a doctor. Thankfully, young, healthy people like my daughter do not typically end up in the ICU due to COVID-19, but my fearless response to her worry turned out to be the right medicine for my *little one*.

Does my experience as a practising physician make me an expert about death and dying? Not really. The real experts on this subject are the dead, but they cannot tell us much. Lucky for us, there are a few exceptions. In Orthodoxy we venerate numerous saints who joyfully died for something far better than this life, and some even encouraged their beloved children to suffer martyrdom for Christ, like Saint Sophia. Their love for Him surpassed their fear of death or their fear of losing a loved one. We also know of miracles of individuals who were raised back from the dead, and some of us have heard personal testimonials or anecdotes of individuals who claim to have died and returned to this life after briefly tasting the beauty and joy of the afterlife. All of us love these stories, but few of us, myself included, can picture ourselves in them, as they tend to be the exception rather than the rule. What, therefore, can I offer, as an ordinary and unworthy Orthodox physician, to describe something about death on a more personally experiential level?

I remember intensely fearing death. Even after pronouncing many patients dead on the wards, I panicked at my first wake as I approached my first open casket. Perhaps it was the casket and the mere thought of burial in the ground that frightened me: but when I laid eyes on the lifeless body inside, the body of another doctor, I realized instantly that that was not all of him. The entirety of him included his life-giving soul, which was no longer there in his body. I had always known that but *seeing* it for the first time somehow *seared* it into the memory of my experience. That life had gone somewhere else, and with it went my fear of "six feet under."

There was another time when I had a panic attack as a patient on a hospital gurney while waiting for the orderlies to wheel me into the operating room. Suddenly I thought, "What if I have an out-of-body experience? What if something goes wrong and I die?" I was not ready to meet God. Instead of praying for His mercy, I began desperately bargaining with Him. It did not help. When I arrived in the operating room and got hooked up to the monitor, my panic was betrayed by the clearly audible rapid beeping that everyone could hear. It subsided only when the anaesthetic took over.

At my two-week post-operative appointment, the surgeon asked how I was feeling. I told him the leg felt fine, but for some reason I could not get my act together. I felt exhausted and unmotivated, as if the life had been sucked out of me. Even my eyes looked empty and lifeless in the mirror. The surgeon said, "Don't worry about it. This is normal. It is post-operative depression because you handed over your life and your control into the hands of others who could make mistakes. It'll pass in a couple of weeks." And it did, which means it *was* "normal."

"Wow," I thought, "I must remember this in my practice."

The next time I needed surgery, I found myself staring at the ceiling of the operating room, again wondering about all the possible outcomes. This time, I resisted giving into fear and bargaining. Instead, I gave my control and myself completely over to God, glorifying Him for all things, even and especially for the imminent procedure. Gratitude felt joyous and freeing, and there was no post-op depression afterwards.

When I contemplate my death, which I find myself doing increasingly as the years pass, my mind does not automatically take me back to those surgical experiences. It takes me back to those times I was giving birth to one of my children. I was not actually dying, of course, but it felt as though I was. Each birthing experience differed from the others, but what stayed the same was what I did not desire—the excruciating pain and an audience. Despite the pain, I still chose natural birth to reduce the risk of complications. Under no circumstances, however, did I desire an audience—those well-meaning family members, witnessing my pain, comparing it to theirs when they had children, offering advice, and cheering me along, as if I were performing an athletic feat. Except for the presence of my husband, who suffered along with me, and the seasoned nurse or doctor, who understood, I preferred privacy. I sought aloneness.

Enduring labour always brought me face to face with the Fall of Humanity. The agonizing curse of labour felt too humbling and humiliating to share, even with those who had already experienced it and meant well. Labour pains entered human history along with Death, which is a blessing from our all-merciful God. Without death, there can be no end to sin and no new Life in Paradise. However, it is a hard and difficult blessing. It reminds me of the joke: *Everybody wants to go to Heaven, but nobody wants to die.* Labour is a type of death, which births new life. Therefore, those birthing pains, those mini deaths that brought the lives of my children into my own life, were both personal and sacred. That is why I did it again and again. My love for my children, even before their conception, surpassed my fears of pain and death. After risking my life to help create new ones, at no time would I wish to see my children mess up their own lives (with panic-stricken COVID-19 measures, for instance) to save mine.

However, I think the main reason I craved aloneness during labour was so I could focus, undistracted, on the task at hand. The long hours of painful labour forced me to reconcile with God and resolve my anger over Eve's curse. For that, I needed every ounce of spiritual strength I could muster. I had no energy or interest in performing, to preclude disappointing anyone or to mitigate the anxieties of amateur labour coach so-and-so next to me, when what I really needed was to come out of that agonizing trial on the right side of Faith.

I imagine dying the same way. The more I think about it, the more I *prefer* to die alone, or at least inconspicuously. Should the Lord bless me with the opportunity for Holy Confession, Holy Communion, and having given and received forgiveness, I then imagine aloneness, unburdened from worrying about the needs of anyone around me, while I prepare to meet my Maker. I imagine birthing my soul, in a delivery room of sorts, utterly stripped of every last shred of dignity, completely humbled and humiliated by my ravaged body (like Christ on the Cross), but all in the presence of my merciful Saviour for whom my soul yearns, because only He, our Great Physician, can *deliver* it and wash it in His precious blood.

Perhaps that is why every freshly dead corpse I have seen (and I have seen many prior to the work of the embalmer) has a look of awe and joy frozen on its face. Despite the still apparent ravages of the illness that killed them, all these faces are beautiful to behold. They are like windows into paradise that give me great hope for the future.

In our fallen world, we understandably feel afraid. However, on the night of His betrayal, Christ faced the sorrow that our fear of death holds over humanity. Out of His love for us, He willingly died on the Cross; He annihilated Death and He gave new Life to the entire world. His suffering was His *labour* of Love. *O Death, where is thy sting? O Hades, where is thy victory?* (1 Corinthians 15:55). It is gone forever, lost in the glory of His awesome Resurrection.

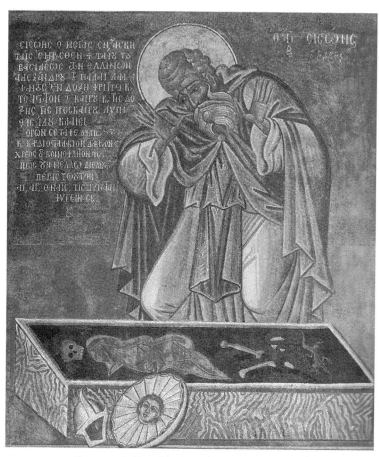

Icon of St. Sisoes at the tomb of
Alexander the Great

CHAPTER 4

Is Cheating Death Worth It? Reflections on Medical Assistance in Dying, Tolstoy, and COVID-19

Irene Polidoulis, MD, CCFP, FCFP

"For a Christian end to our lives, painless, blameless, peaceful, and a good defense before the awesome Judgement Seat of Christ, let us ask of the Lord."

This petition from the Divine Liturgy of St. John Chrysostom shows how important a role both our life and death play in preparing us for eternity. Leo Tolstoy attempts to illustrate this in two great works, despite his own "un-Orthodox" personal beliefs in Jesus of Nazareth as a mere teacher of ethics who was not divine, did not perform miracles, did not rise from the dead, and does not reign in a heavenly kingdom that does not exist.[1]

Perhaps Tolstoy's strictly terrestrial worldview is even more reason for us to appreciate what he offers Christians and the rest of the world through two of his fictional narratives. In *The*

---

1. That anti-Orthodox theology plus the mockery of the Orthodox Divine Liturgy and Orthodox clergy in his final novel, Resurrection, in 1899 led to his public excommunication in 1901 by the Russian Orthodox Church.

Death of Ivan Ilyich, he devotes an entire novella to the main character's sinful life, which he only begins to understand during his escalating inner spiritual battle as he lies dying. In *War and Peace*, Tolstoy's Prince Andrei finally learns to love after he escapes death long enough to forgive betrayal and watch his hated enemy die.

If Prince Andrei and Ivan Ilyich were non-fictional persons alive today, both might have been deprived of those blessings by Medical Assistance in Dying (MAID). Since March 17, 2021, and according to the Criminal Code in Canada, a "mentally competent adult (18 years or older)" may access MAID if he or she satisfies all the following criteria, including but not limited to:

- Having a serious and incurable illness, disease or disability
- Being in an advanced state of irreversible decline in capability
- Experiencing enduring and intolerable suffering as a result of their medical condition
- Being on a course toward the end of life. Death would have to be reasonably foreseeable in all the circumstances of a person's health, but there would not have to be a specific prognosis or prospected time period before death.[2]

The *Criminal Code of Canada* currently prohibits "physicians, nurse practitioners—and those who help them"[3] from administering MAID to patients based solely on a mental

---

2. Bullet points quoted from Department of Justice Canada, "Medical Assistance in Dying": https://www.canada.ca/en/department-justice/news/2016/04/medical-assistance-in-dying.html (Accessed on January 12, 2022).

3. Ibid.

illness. However, the Canadian federal government plans to revisit this exclusion by 2023, making it possible also for mentally ill people to choose MAID instead of suicide.

Once all the criteria are satisfied, MAID becomes as easy as one simple (and expensive) injection to induce a sleep from which one never awakens. The intent is to give the already dying a more *dignified* exit, by avoiding the final ravages of their illness. By expediting their death, the dying person can take more *control* over it. There is also an added *convenience*. The dying can choose to bring their loved ones together at a pre-arranged date and time for their death, instead of burdening them with unexpected, last-minute preparations for travel, funeral arrangements and so on. One can even, if still able, dress oneself in one's funeral attire before receiving the lethal injection. In the case of the Brickendens, the ageing couple was even able to arrange to die *together* so that neither one suffered the loss of the other, while their children watched from the foot of their bed.[4] To a *suffering* individual or a *fearful* individual, a *proud* or a *desperate* individual, MAID can be attractive on many levels.

Does MAID really cheat death, though? Or does it cheat us? It may feel *empowering* to think that we are cheating death somehow by circumventing the agony of dying, but modern medicine with its palliative care options, has made it possible to eliminate physical pain, or at least to diminish it to a significant degree. If there is psychological or spiritual pain, this is what the Church calls a *lack of peace*. This type of agony sometimes pushes to the surface of one's consciousness the ugly parts of one's life—the parts one would otherwise

---

4. "Medically assisted death allows couple married almost 73 years to die together," The Globe and Mail, April 1, 2018.

ignore and forget—forcing a person to reconcile within, with others, and with God in the form of *repentance*.

In *War and Peace*, Prince Andrei Bolkonsky was a bitter and angry man when he became mortally wounded in 1812, fighting Napoleon's Grand Army of France on the field of Borodino. He ardently hated the man who had seduced his fiancée into an elopement, but he hated her even more for her childish infatuation with Anatole and her betrayal of Prince Andrei's own honourable love for her. Although the elopement had been discovered and intercepted, and Natasha suffered tremendous shame and remorse afterwards, Prince Andrei could not forgive her. He broke off their engagement and his promises to her, and in so doing, became a disenchanted and broken man. Such was the condition of his heart when he was severely wounded in battle. His doctor, knowing there was no hope for his survival, felt regret when the prince partially recovered, "for if he did not die now, he would do so a little later with greater suffering."[5] Prince Andrei's sufferings, however, become a transformative blessing.

After he was carried off the battlefield, Prince Andrei was set on a table in a dressing station to have his wound examined and dressed. On the table next to him, another wounded soldier was undergoing a horrifying leg amputation. "In the miserable, sobbing, shattered creature whose leg had just been amputated, he [Prince Andrei] recognized Anatole Kuragin," the man who had seduced Natasha. Suddenly, Tolstoy narrates:

---

5. All quotations of *War and Peace* are from Rosemary Edmunds' translation, Penguin, 2009.

his soul awoke to a love and tenderness for her which were stronger and more pulsing with life than they had ever been . . . [He] remembered everything and a passionate pity and love for this man welled up in his happy heart. [He] could no longer restrain himself and wept tender compassionate tears for his fellow men, for himself and for their errors and his own.

The dying prince thought to himself, "Sympathy, love for our brothers, for those who love us and for those who hate us, love of our enemies—yes, the love that God preached on earth, that Princess Maria [his sister] tried to teach me and I did not understand . . .

"Yes—love. But not that love which loves for something, to gain something or because of something, but the love I knew for the first time when, dying, I saw my enemy and yet loved him. I experienced the love which is the very essence of the soul, the love which requires no object. And I feel that blessed feeling now too. To love one's neighbours, to love one's enemies, to love everything—to love God in all His manifestations. Human love serves to love those dear to us but to love one's enemies we need divine love. And that is why I knew such joy when I felt I loved that man. What became of him? Is he alive? . . . Human love may turn to hatred, but divine love cannot change. Nothing, not even death can destroy it. It is the very nature of the soul. Yet how many people have I hated in my life? And of them all, none did I love and hate as much as her." And he vividly pictured Natasha to himself, not as he had pictured her in the past with her charms only, which gave him such delight, but for the first time imagining her soul. And he understood her feelings, her suffering, her shame, and remorse. Now, for the first time, he realized all the cruelty of his rejection of her, the cruelty of breaking with her. "If only I might see her once more. Just once to look into those eyes and say . . ."

When he came to himself Natasha, the veritable living Natasha, whom of all people he most longed to love with the new, pure, divine love that had been revealed to him, was on her knees before him . . . [She] knelt . . . gazing at him with frightened eyes and restraining her sobs . . . Prince Andrei fetched a sigh of relief, smiled, and held out his hand . . .

It seems providential that Prince Andrei survived a shell blast that should have instantly killed him, and then witnessed the brutal amputation of his sworn enemy, Anatole, followed by the bitter remorse of the woman his enemy had seduced. Instead of feeling vindicated, the synchronous experience of his own suffering and dying engendered compassion for his enemy and his fiancée and turned his hatred of them into love. The good doctor, drenched in the blood of the wounded while immersed in saving their lives, could not know any of this. Naturally, he wished Prince Andrei a quick death to spare him more physical suffering. Tolstoy, however, who knew the back story (because he wrote it) also knew that a *quick* death would have cheated Prince Andrei from a *good* death, a death that would teach the prince (and the reader) the power of forgiveness and the beauty of divine love.

This was also the case in *The Death of Ivan Ilyich*. According to Tolstoy, "*the past history of Ivan Ilyich's life was most simple and ordinary and most terrible.*" [6] It was most terrible, not because of the way he died (which until the very end was also terrible) but because of the way he lived, which was how most people lived within his social circle. And yet, Ivan Ilyich was not a *bad* person. He

> was an intelligent, lively, pleasant, and decent man . . . educated in law school . . . [and] strict in fulfilling what he considered his duty [which was] all that was so considered by highly placed people. He was not ingratiating . . . but from the earliest age he [was] drawn . . . to the most highly placed people in society . . . adopting their manners, their views of life, and . . . establishing friendly relations with them . . .

Ivan Ilyich had opportunities to repent of his sins early in his life, but he did not.

> In law school he had committed acts which had formerly seemed to him of great vileness and had inspired a feeling of self-loathing . . . but subsequently, seeing that such acts were also committed by highly placed people and were not considered bad, he, without really thinking them good, forgot all about them and was not troubled in the least by the memory of them . . .
>
> Even after law school . . . he had been given to sensuality and vanity . . . there was a liaison in the provinces with one of the ladies . . . there was also a milliner [hat maker]; there were drinking parties . . . and little trips to a remote back street after supper; there was also subservience to his superior and even to his superior's wife; but it all

---

6. All quotations of *The Death of Ivan Ilyich & Other Stories* are from Richard Pevear and Larissa Volokhonsky's translation, Knopf, 2009.

bore such a lofty tone of propriety that it could not be called by any bad words . . . It was all done with clean hands, in clean shirts, with French words, and above all in the highest society . . . with the approval of highly placed people . . ."

And so, Ivan Ilyich never felt the need to trouble himself with change or repentance, something which his social circle did not practice or even think about. Although he never abused his power as an examining magistrate, Ivan Ilyich continued making an idol of himself and of the high society whose approval he always sought, devoting his life to every elegance and pleasure he could afford and consciously putting on those airs he felt suited his station in life.

He sought only to pass his life easily and pleasantly. For a while, this worked out well. Even his marriage was very pleasant at first, until his wife began to experience the discomforts of pregnancy and new motherhood, which revealed to her the callous selfishness of her husband. The more she tried to solicit his support and assistance with her difficulties, the more he felt her entreaties disrupted "the pleasantness and decency of life," and the more he ignored her. He spent less and less time with his family, devoting himself increasingly to his work and to his friends. Soon, he and his wife were developing an ever-deepening animosity for one another. Even this did not bother him, however, provided there was no quarreling and he always had something pleasant with which to occupy himself.

After seventeen years of a troubled marriage that he did his best to ignore, Ivan Ilyich was still relatively young at 45 when he developed an ache in his side. At first, he ignored it, just as he had ignored his wife. But the ache kept growing, forcing him to experience a mounting unpleasantness, which progressively disrupted his chosen lifestyle whether he liked it or not. First, he had to seek out doctors and take medications. Then, the pain interfered with his ability to work, ultimately forcing him to stop work altogether. Card games, which he loved, initially distracted him from the pain, but, eventually, he could not enjoy those either. Eating also became problematic, followed by sitting with company, and he began needing to leave the room to lie down in private.

This gradual withdrawal peeved his family, particularly his wife who had grown so accustomed to his passive-aggressiveness that she believed him to be purposely behaving this way, just to spite her. Instead of giving her husband the sympathy he craved, she even blamed him for his illness. Unfortunately, Ivan Ilyich could not see that he had brought this treatment from her upon himself, because he had treated her the same way.

While the pleasantries of life for his family went on without him, Ivan Ilyich made more frequent visits to more doctors, took increasing doses of opium and morphine, and began to experience a heightening realization that he might actually be dying. After eight weeks of decline, he became bed ridden, while bearing the humiliation of a male servant having to change his clothing and carry him from place to place. By the time his doctors and his family realized that he was, indeed, dying, Ivan Ilyich's main torment changed. It was no longer the physical pain and the resentment he felt towards others for living life without him; it was now everyone's "lie" that he was merely ill and not dying. He was often a hair's breadth away from shouting, "Stop lying!" But he never had the courage to do it. "The dreadful, terrible act of his dying . . . was reduced by all those around him to the

level of an accidental unpleasantness, partly an indecency
. . . in the name of that very 'decency' he had served all his
life . . . "

Ten weeks into his illness, everything became too much for
him to bear. He "stopped holding himself back and wept like
a child . . . over his helplessness, over his terrible loneliness,
over the cruelty of people, over the cruelty of God, over the
absence of God."

> Finally, Ivan Ilyich prayed: "Why have You done all
> this? Why have You brought me here? Why, why do you
> torment me so terribly?"
>
> "What do you want?" was the first clear idea that he
> heard.
>
> "What? Not to suffer. To live," he replied.
>
> "To live? To live how?" asked the voice of his soul.
>
> "Yes, to live as I lived before: nicely, pleasantly."
>
> "As you lived before, nicely and pleasantly?" asked
> the voice. He started to remember the best moments of
> his pleasant life, but strangely, all that had seemed like
> joys dissolved away, turning into something worthless
> and vile. Only his childhood seemed right to him. The
> further away from childhood he remembered, the more
> worthless and dubious were his joys. His climb in public
> opinion was proportional to the downhill decline of the
> remainder of his life. Then, the thought "Maybe I did
> not live as I should have" suddenly came into his head,
> but this made no sense to him at first because he had
> done "everything one ought to," according to social
> expectations.
>
> "What do you want now then?" his soul challenged.
> "To live? To live how? To live as you live in court, when

the usher proclaims: 'Court is in session!' Court is in session, court is in session . . . Here is the court!"

"But I'm not guilty!" Ivan Ilyich shouted angrily. Again, he recalled all the correctness of his life and drove away the strange thought.

Another two weeks of agony went by before Ivan Ilyich reconsidered that perhaps he had, in fact, not lived rightly and this time he was able to see that this was so, both in himself and in his social circle. He saw "a terrible, vast deception concealing both life and death. This consciousness increased his physical sufferings tenfold." He felt desperate. It made him hate both his family and everyone in his social class. When his wife called a priest for communion, this eased him only momentarily. For the next three days, Ivan Ilyich howled horrifically and spent every ounce of energy he had left thrashing from side to side, as though he were physically trying to push away all the horror of his life that had been revealed to him. By the end of the third day, he calmed down and said to himself, "Yes, it was *all* not right . . . but never mind. I can, I can *do* 'right.' But what *is* 'right'?"

Just then, his young son entered the room, grabbed his father's hand and weeping, kissed it. His wife also came in, her face tear stained and desperate. For the first time, Ivan Ilyich realized he had been tormenting them and he felt sorry for them. For the first time, he asked them to forgive him, and suddenly his torment resolved. "'How good and how simple,' he thought . . . 'And death? Where is it?'. . . There was no more fear because there was no more death. Instead of death there was light. 'So that's it!' he suddenly said aloud. 'What joy!'" For those around him, his apparent physical agony went on for two more hours, but for Ivan Ilyich, whose sufferings had ceased the moment he experienced Truth, the time passed in an instant.

"'It's finished!' someone said over him."

"'Death is finished,' he said to himself. 'It is no more,'" and Ivan Ilyich took in his final breath but his first eternally happy and peaceful one.

Many of us can relate to Ivan Ilyich, who devoted his entire life to making an idol of himself and his lifestyle. We can also relate to at least some of his sins, which seduced and deluded him under the guise of "decency"—his vanity, posturing, selfishness, shallowness, pride, worldliness, sensuality, hypocrisy, enmity, and idolatry to name a few. Because he was not as bad as some and kept himself within the law, Ivan Ilyich had successfully deluded himself about the "decency" of his life to the degree of spiritual blindness, much like the Pharisees at the time of Christ. And yet, God did not give up on Ivan Ilyich. Knowing how far gone he was but not hopelessly so, He blessed Ivan Ilyich with as much suffering as he needed *to open the eyes of this blind man* (as they were closing in death) to the truth of his terrible life, leading him to repentance, salvation, and joy. When the fruit of Ivan Ilyich's soul finally became ripe and ready to be transplanted into the eternal garden of paradise, only then did our loving God take it there.

Tolstoy's world (and ours as well) was filled with "decent" Ivan Ilyiches whose main goal in life was the pursuit of pleasure and ease, even amongst those who practised a form of Christianity. This story, therefore, explains the purpose behind the torment of forgotten or unrecognized sin.

This type of torment becomes a blessing when it leads to repentance.

A classic real-life example is the death of the penitent thief on the cross next to Christ. His death was not "painless, blameless or peaceful." It was agonizing and shameful torture, but because the Lord knew the condition of his heart, this man was blessed with the experience of crucifixion next to Christ as a final but most profound opportunity to confess his sins. That confession became the salvific "Christian end" to the life of the thief when Christ said to him, "Today, you shall be with Me in Paradise." (Luke 23:43)

On the other hand, Prince Andrei's story successfully drives home the extremes of betrayal, hatred, love, repentance, and forgiveness that often battle it out in the hearts and minds of those who strive for spiritual growth and righteousness. It took a mortal physical wound to help Prince Andrei reach this salvific spiritual level.

Leo Tolstoy, the non-believer but literary master, managed somehow, perhaps providentially, to depict in the spiritual transformation of his characters Prince Andrei and Ivan Ilyich the purpose of suffering, the mystery of death, and the nature of God's divine love. We Orthodox Christians believe unabashedly that since Christ condescended to death on the cross, He will also do whatever *else* it takes to save us, individualizing our dying experience according to the spiritual needs of each one of us. "O Death, where is thy sting? O Hades, where is thy victory?" (1 Corinthians 15:55) does not only refer to Christ's one-time destruction of Hades, but also to His Life-offering faithful presence as each of us dies. He persistently and tirelessly knocks on the door of our hearts, even to the very end of our earthly lives, if we have not "lived as [we] should have." Had Tolstoy's characters not died the way they did, they would have been deprived of the most profound experiences of their lives (their salvation), and we would have been deprived of the priceless lessons they learned.

We all hope for a "painless, blameless and peaceful ending," but if we do not live as we should, God, in His unfathomable loving-kindness may grant us enough difficulty in dying to teach us the lessons we resisted learning while alive and well. This is not by way of punishment, but by way of lovingly helping us truly repent, to ensure that our own unique experience of death transforms us and transports us from the land of the dying to the realm of the living.

There are many examples of difficult deaths that opened the gates of paradise. The holy martyrs who lived for Christ, often suffered, some by way of physical torture, others through spiritual battles, and still others by rejecting the pleasures of this world, to name a few examples. What would have happened to them if they took the easy way out—if MAID had intercepted their physical and spiritual struggles? What can happen to us if we allow MAID to intercept our own dying process? For many, as in the case of the pleasure-seeking Ivan Ilyiches of the world, *death* affords the *last* opportunity for repentance and salvation. Similarly, every crisis in *life*—a grave illness, a war, a plague—becomes a blessed opportunity for a return to the narrow path of salvific living.

On the one hand, MAID undermines the sanctity of life and a salvific death by indulging inordinate desires for dignity, control, and convenience among those who wish to orchestrate their own deaths. On the other hand, the present COVID-19 crisis has plunged many "decent" people into such a vortex of extreme panic and an all-consuming fear of death from the corona virus, that they seem to have lost all hope and confidence in the providence of the loving Son of God, who suffered and died for our sins, conquered death, and promises eternal life in the kingdom of heaven for those who love Him and abide by His teachings. In stark contrast to Tolstoy's Ivan Ilych and Prince Andrei, these people try to cling to physical life on earth at any cost, even by avoiding the Holy Mysteries and the liturgical services of the Holy Orthodox Church for fear of "catching COVID-19."

For love of God and neighbour, we should do all we can to alleviate the suffering of any human condition and to mitigate the effects of any war, plague, or other crisis. However, playing God by hastening death through MAID does not cheat death. It only cheats the dying out of eternal life. Similarly, losing hope in divine providence during a pandemic or other crisis is not "safe." It, too, cheats—the survivors out of salvific living *"and a good defense before the awesome Judgement Seat of Christ."*

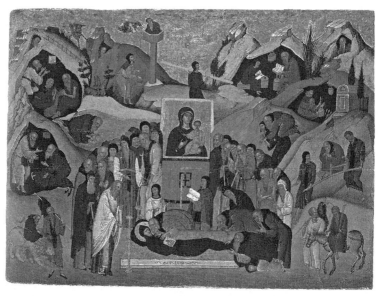

Icon of the burial of St. Ephraim the Syrian,
surrounded by his monks

CHAPTER 5

The COVID-19 Panic: A Lost Opportunity for Palliative Care

Irene Polidoulis, MD, CCFP, FCFP

Death has always been a part of life. It has always been the expectation that people living in nursing homes or with a life-limiting illness will eventually die. Part of the natural order of things is for the oldest, the weakest, and the most ailing members of society to experience the greatest proportion of deaths at any given time. Before the advances in modern medicine and the proliferation of hospitals for the masses, the passage from life to death usually occurred at home, in the presence of caring loved ones, and sometimes with visits from the local doctor and the parish priest. Today, we call this palliative care.

In 2018, two years before the COVID-19 Pandemic, Canadian Minister of Health, Ginette Petitpas Taylor, wrote this inspiring introduction to the *Framework on Palliative Care in Canada.*[1]

---

1. Framework on Palliative Care in Canada, Health Canada, Dec 2018 (modified July 12, 2019): https://www.canada.ca/en/health-canada/services/health-care-system/reports-publications/palliative-care/framework-palliative-care-canada.html#rem (All websites in this chapter accessed on January 24, 2022).

Many Canadians find it difficult to discuss death, dying and end-of-life care with their loved ones and health care providers. We tend to avoid these conversations out of **fear and pain**.[2] *Yet, these topics are important to the well-being of dying people and their families. Encouraging Canadians to have honest and informed conversations about death and end-of-life planning can alleviate stress, anxiety and help to ensure that Canadians have* **the death that they wish***.*

Over time, our experience of death and dying has evolved alongside changing causes of death, care and supports, and cultural and social customs. The provision of palliative care has also evolved as a practice that seeks to relieve suffering and **improve the quality of living and dying** *for Canadians and their families. However, we know* **we have more to do** *to improve* **person-centred care** *and* **equitable access***, so that every Canadian has the best possible quality of life right up to the end of their lives.*

Over the course of the summer of 2018, officials from Health Canada heard many stories of dedication and commitment about people living with life-limiting illness, caregivers, volunteers, and health care providers. There were, however, also stories pointing to significant **gaps in awareness** *and* **understanding** *of, and* **access** *to, palliative care across Canada.*

The message from these conversations was clear: the **wishes and needs of Canadians nearing the end of life must be at the centre** *of our approaches to care. It is critical that their cultural values and personal preferences be voiced, understood and respected when discussing care plans and treatment*

---

2. Boldface added in this chapter for emphasis.

options. This message inspired and influenced the **Framework on Palliative Care in Canada**...

The Honourable Ginette Petitpas Taylor, P.C., M.P.
Minister of Health

According to the *Framework on Palliative Care in Canada*,[3] palliative care is defined as an approach to care that reduces suffering and improves the quality of life of people (and their families) of all ages (including children) with life-limiting illness. It does this by providing:

- Pain and symptom management,
- Psychological, social, emotional, spiritual, and practical support, and
- Support for caregivers, both during the illness and after the death of their loved one.[4]

"Palliative care" first emerged in Canada in the mid-1970's, first as a medical specialty, primarily serving hospitalized cancer patients. Since then, the scope of palliative care has expanded to include *all* people, both children and adults, living with any type of life-limiting illness. Owing to our aging population, the demand for palliative care continues to grow in Canada[5] and throughout the world.

---

3. *Framework on Palliative Care in Canada*, Health Canada, Dec 2018 (modified July 12, 2019): https://www.canada.ca/content/dam/hc-sc/documents/services/health-care-system/reports-publications/palliative-care/framework-palliative-care-canada/framework-palliative-care-canada.pdf.

4. https://www.canada.ca/en/health-canada/services/health-care-system/reports-publications/palliative-care/framework-palliative-care-canada.html#p1.1.

5. Lee Sharkey, Belinda Loring, Melanie Cowan, Leanne riley, Eric L Krakauer, "National palliative care capacities around the world: Results

Palliative care is not exclusive of other types of health care. Communities can provide it in conjunction with other treatment plans, in a variety of settings (such as the home, the hospice, the nursing home, the hospital), and by a variety of health care providers (doctors, nurses, nurse practitioners, pharmacists, social workers, occupational/speech therapists, and psychological, religious, or spiritual counsellors).

According to the World Health Organization (WHO), the definition of palliative care[6] includes:

1. Effective "relief from pain and other distressing symptoms"
2. An affirmation of life while regarding "dying as a normal process"
3. Neither hastening nor postponing death
4. Integrating "the psychological and spiritual aspects of patient care"
5. Offering "a support system to help patients live as actively as possible until death"
6. Offering "a support system to help the family cope during the patient's illness and in their own bereavement"
7. Using a team approach to address the needs of patients and their families, including bereavement counseling, if indicated
8. Enhancing "quality of life" and favorably influencing the course of illness

from the World Health Organization Noncommunicable Disease Country Capacity Survey," *Palliative Medicine* (January 2018) 32:1, 106-113. DOI: 10.1177/0269216317716060. EPUB (July 5, 2017): https://pubmed.ncbi.nlm.nih.gov/28677988/.

6. *Framework on Palliative Care in Canada*, Health Canada, Dec 2018, modified July 12, 2019: http://www.who.int/cancer/palliative/definition/en/.

9. Providing palliative care "early in the course of illness, in conjunction with other therapies that are intended to prolong life, such as chemotherapy or radiation therapy," including "those investigations needed to better understand and manage distressing clinical complications"

The Journal of Palliative Medicine Special Report[7] expressed the benefits of palliative care in 2012. Patients with chronic progressive diseases (such as congestive heart failure, chronic obstructive pulmonary disease, HIV/AIDS, or cancer) can develop severe physical, psychosocial, and spiritual symptoms before death. However, there is compelling evidence that palliative care is beneficial in reducing much of this suffering, as well as the psychosocial and spiritual or existential distress experienced by the families of these patients.[8]

The Canadian *Framework on Palliative Care* describes *Ten Guiding Principles* in Palliative Care:[9]

1. Palliative care is person- and family-centred.
2. Death, dying, grief, and bereavement are part of life.
3. Caregivers are both providers and recipients of care.

---

7. Sharon Tapper, "Special Report: New Frontiers for Palliative Care: Centre for Medicare and Medicaid Innovation," *Journal of Palliative Medicine* (July 31, 2012) Vol 15 No 8 pp 844-845: https://doi.org/10.1089/jpm.2012.0090. 6 *Framework on Palliative Care in Canada*, Health Canada, Dec 2018, modified July 12, 2019: http://www.who.int/cancer/palliative/definition/en/.

8. Deborah Cook, Graeme Rocker and Daren Heyland, "Enhancing the Quality of End of Life Care in Canada," *Canadian Medical Association Journal* (Nov 05, 2013) 185 (16) pp 1383-1384; DOI: https://doi.org/10.1503/cmaj.130716.

9. *Framework on Palliative Care in Canada*, Health Canada, Dec 2018, modified July 12, 2019: https://www.canada.ca/en/health-canada/services/health-care-system/reports-publications/palliative-care/framework-palliative-care-canada.html#p2.2.

4. Palliative care is integrated and holistic.
5. Access to palliative care is equitable.
6. Palliative care recognizes and values the diversity of Canada and its peoples.
7. Palliative care services are valued, understood, and adequately resourced.
8. Palliative care is high quality and Evidence-Based.
9. **Palliative care improves quality of life.**
10. Palliative care is a shared responsibility.

The three principles in boldface are especially relevant to our topic and worth discussing in more detail.

The first of these is that palliative care is meant to be ***person- and family-centred***. This means that the person receiving care and his or her family are at the centre of the decision making, placing *that person's* values and wishes at the forefront of treatment considerations. The voices of people living with life-limiting illness and their families are sought and respected. The health care provider(s) alone do not decide palliative care treatment plans. Providers develop plans *in partnership* with the person living with life-limiting illness and the family, while respecting their values and their cultural and spiritual preferences.

The second guiding principle is that ***death, dying, grief, and bereavement are a part of life***. This requires a cultural *shift* in how we talk about death and dying—a shift *away from* fear and avoidance and *towards* acceptance and understanding of the dying process, what palliative care really is and how it can *positively* impact people's lives. Integrating palliative care at the *initial stages* of life-limiting illness facilitates this cultural shift by supporting honest and meaningful discussions with those affected and with their families and caregivers, regarding care that is consistent with their values and preferences.

The third guiding principle is that palliative care reduces suffering and ***improves quality of life*** for people with life-limiting illness and their families. This principle makes palliative care appropriate for people of *all* ages, including children, with *any* life-limiting illness, and at *any point* in their illness trajectory, even when death is expected several years down the road. Whereas palliative care used to be delivered predominantly in hospitals by specialists, ideally it should be available in any setting—including the home, retirement home, nursing home, or other setting of choice—and by all types of health care providers, including family physicians, nurses, chaplains, and others. Whereas palliative care was available almost exclusively in the last weeks of life, ideally it should be offered immediately upon a diagnosis of a life-limiting illness. Whereas palliative care used to be discussed only after all other medical interventions were exhausted, ideally it should be discussed in conjunction with other appropriate medical interventions at the outset of treatment. In cases of a life-limiting illness of any duration, treatment plans should always include palliative care to improve and maximize quality of life through to the end of life.

In my experience, palliative care has been one of the most rewarding aspects of medical practice. Palliative care-giving from loved ones can create treasured memories, profound intimacy, and a deep sense of accomplishment. Personal relationships can become cemented and grow, providing tremendous comfort to families in the grieving process. However, the nature of some deaths may exceed a caregiver's ability to cope while caring for a loved one at home. This often results in admission to a hospice or a hospital's palliative care unit in the final months, weeks, or days of life. That trend underscores the importance of institutional initiatives, not to prolong life artificially but to improve end-of-life care while still avoiding the "medicalization of death." This approach beyond the home continues to offer holistic family-centred care as well as options for ongoing assessment and treatment of symptoms.[10]

To recap what Health Minister Ginette Petitpas Taylor wrote, "*We know we have more to do to improve person-centred care and equitable access, so that every Canadian has the best possible quality of life right up to the end of their lives.*"[11] This statement is not only true of Canada, but of most countries around the world, since only a minority (37%) have an operational national policy for palliative care.[12] As is the case with most countries, the palliative care gap means that access to palliative care is uneven across Canada both by location and population.

We need to ensure that palliative care support and services are available to all those who need them, regardless of where they live or their personal characteristics. We need to include caregivers, who still tend to be on the periphery of the health

---

10. Deborah Cook, Graeme Rocker and Daren Heyland, "Enhancing the Quality of End of Life Care in Canada," *Canadian Medical Association Journal* (Nov 05, 2013) 185 (16) pp 1383-1384: https://doi.org/10.1503/cmaj.130716.

11. *Framework on Palliative Care in Canada*, Health Canada, Dec 2018, modified July 12, 2019, "Remarks from Minister Ginette Petitpas Taylor, P.C., M.P.": https://www.canada.ca/en/health-canada/services/health-care-system/reports-publications/palliative-care/framework-palliative-care-canada.html#rem.

12. Lee Sharkey, Belinda Loring, Melanie Cowan, Leanne riley, Eric L Krakauer, "National palliative care capacities around the world: Results from the World Health Organization Noncommunicable Disease Country Capacity Survey," *Palliative Medicine* (January 2018) 32:1, 106-113: https://pubmed.ncbi.nlm.nih.gov/28677988/.

care team, as a central and consulted part of the decision-making or care-planning process. In addition, there are no Canadian national standards for data collection or use and few person-centred outcome or experience measures. Furthermore, there is still insufficient support for Canadian research specific to palliative care.[13] Since that is probably true for most other countries, it must change there, too.

According to the World Health Organization, it is estimated that only 14% of patients who need palliative care receive it.[14] In a 2013 study published in the Canadian Medical Association Journal (CMAJ), 278 acutely ill elderly Canadians with advanced chronic disease and their families were interviewed in twelve hospitals. Over three-quarters of these patients had thought about end-of-life care and had discussed it with a family member, but rarely with a member of their health care team, such as a doctor or a nurse. For only 30% of these patients did the hospital medical record reflect their preferences for less-intensive management at the end of life. In the other 70% who preferred less-intensive end of life management, their medical records included plans for full resuscitation and technologic support in the event of a life-threatening illness in hospital.[15]

---

13. Deborah Cook, Graeme Rocker and Daren Heyland, "Enhancing the Quality of End of Life Care in Canada," *Canadian Medical Association Journal* (Nov 05, 2013) 185 (16) pp 1383-1384; DOI: https://doi.org/10.1503/cmaj.130716.

14. World Health Organization, "Palliative Care": https://who.int/health-topics/palliative-care.

15. Deborah Cook, Graeme Rocker and Daren Heyland, "Enhancing the Quality of End of Life Care in Canada," *Canadian Medical Association Journal* (Nov 05, 2013) 185 (16) pp 1383-1384; DOI: https://doi.org/10.1503/cmaj.130716.

We can avoid this unfortunate scenario through **Advanced Care Planning**, which is an organized process of communication to help patients and their families understand, reflect upon, and discuss their goals, values, and beliefs for future health care decisions. This is especially important if the ailing person loses the ability to communicate. Personalized, compassionate, and culturally sensitive end-of-life care is everyone's right, but making it a reality requires more intense efforts by citizens, families, patients, providers, and policymakers working together toward this especially important goal.[16] Advanced Care Planning is not just for those in palliative care or those with a life-limiting illness. It can apply to anyone and at any stage of their life, who wishes to clarify the care they desire in the event of a life-threatening or life-limiting illness, should they lose the ability to communicate.[17]

More recent data published in September 2018 by the Canadian Institute for Health Information (CIHI) revealed that even those who manage to get palliative care in Canada still tend to get it late, and that far too many dying patients are still shuffled around between home, hospitals, and nursing homes in their final days. While 75% of Canadians preferred to die at home, only about 15% had access to palliative home care services and did die at home. According to the Globe and Mail in Toronto, therefore, Canada is not a good place to die.[18] Again, if this is true of Canada, it is probably true of

---

16. Ibid.

17. Ibid.

18. Globe and Mail, https://www.theglobeandmail.com/canada/article-new-data-show-canada-ranks-among-worlds-worst-for-ltc-deaths/.

most countries around the world, and it has been tragically true during the panic over COVID-19.

According to Statistics Canada, 282, 890 Canadians died in the July 2018 - June 2019 pre-pandemic year.[19] In the Framework on Palliative Care in Canada, updated in 2019, 90% of these people, about 254, 600 Canadians, died of a chronic, life-limiting illness such as heart disease, organ failure, cancer, dementia, or frailty. Because of Canada's ageing population, the number and proportion of deaths due to chronic illness is projected to increase further over time.[20] According to CIHI data, 75% of that 90% would have preferred to die at home but only 15% actually did, meaning that 60%, or 152, 760 Canadians, did not receive the palliative care and/or the home death they wished for just prior to the COVID-19 pandemic.[21] How do we understand these figures in a COVID-19 environment?

By January 2022, roughly 32,500 Canadians of all ages had died with a diagnosis of COVID-19,[22] with about 25,200 of these COVID-19 deaths[23] (77.5%) occurring in people 70+ years of age. If, according to Canadian statistics, 90% of Canadians died of a chronic, life-limiting illness in 2018-2019, one may reasonably argue that 90% of the 25,200 Canadians 70+ years of age, (or 22,680) who died with COVID-19, also had at least one life-limiting illness.

19. https://www.statista.com/statistics/443061/number-of-deaths-in-canada/.

20. *Framework on Palliative Care in Canada*, Health Canada, Dec 2018, modified July 12, 2019, "Death and Dying in Canada."

21. Globe and Mail, https://www.theglobeandmail.com/canada/article-new-data-show-canada-ranks-among-worlds-worst-for-ltc-deaths/.

22. https://health-infobase.canada.ca/covid-19/epidemiological-summa-ry-covid-19-cases.html#a1.

23. https://www.statista.com/statistics/1228632/number-covid-deaths-canada-by-age/.

According to CIHI, about 75% of these people would have preferred to die at home but only 15% did, which means an estimated 60% (13,608 of Canadian elderly) died, instead, in hospital, many of them on life support. This represents approximately 42% of Canadians, who have thus far died of COVID-19 in hospital, instead of at home with palliative care measures, as they would have wished. This already significant estimate does not include those COVID-19 victims under the age of 70, who may have also preferred palliative care.

If all who would have preferred to die at home could have done so, our Canadian hospitals would never have been at risk of over capacity due to this pandemic. I do realize that these numbers are broad strokes, but this is the best conservative estimate I can make at this time, since research is still on-going, and there are no Canadian national standards for data collection or use and few person-centred outcome or experience measures in palliative care.[24]

Life-limiting illness is not as simple as it sounds. Many do not realize that often, it is not the life-limiting illness itself that ultimately claims the life of the individual. Rather, it is the complications arising from that illness. After the life-limiting illness has sufficiently weakened the body, the ultimate cause of death is frequently some type of infection, such as a viral or bacterial pneumonia, a urinary tract infection, or even the common cold. Bacterial pneumonia was the final straw that claimed the life of my father-in-law who was palliatively hospitalized for stage IV prostate cancer. Other types of

24. Deborah Cook, Graeme Rocker and Daren Heyland, "Enhancing the Quality of End of Life Care in Canada," *Canadian Medical Association Journal* (Nov 05, 2013) 185 (16) pp 1383-1384; DOI: https://doi.org/10.1503/cmaj.130716.

common infections frequently hasten the demise of other seriously ill people, including COVID-19.

Treatment of *any* infection near the end of life is inappropriate in palliative care, since it prolongs the dying process and the dying person's suffering, something that is contrary to the third point in the WHO definition of palliative care outlined above. Allowing an infection to hasten the demise of those near the end of life is the acceptable and humane ***high standard*** of medical practice. It would have been unthinkable to prescribe antibiotics to my dying father-in-law; and yet, many who wished to die peacefully and with dignity during the pandemic, ended up on a ventilator in intensive care because of an infection with COVID-19.

After those deaths with (and not necessarily because of) COVID-19, what was the cause of death that was written on their death certificate? Was it their life-limiting illness(es), or was it COVID-19 alone? To record only COVID-19 while not including the life-limiting illness(es) would be akin to writing down "pneumonia" in the case of my father-in-law, without including "stage IV prostate cancer." When we, his family, talk about his death, we never say that he died of pneumonia, but that he died of prostate cancer, because he never would have died of pneumonia if he did not first have terminal prostate cancer. Unfortunately, this type of long-established reporting standard did not seem to prevail in the case of COVID-19, (at least not in the media) where every individual's life-limiting illness was upstaged by the panic of the SARS-CoV-2 virus. If a diagnosis of COVID-19 has replaced what should have been a different, or at least an additional primary cause of death in our data collection, it will bias important future research and policy making in a potentially harmful way.

Equally unfortunate is that the COVID-19 deaths of those who preferred quiet, palliative care instead of aggressive or invasive, life-saving care, made sensational front-page news for weeks on end, accompanied by horrifying descriptions like "drowning in their lung fluids" and "dying alone" in the company of "staff," instead of their loved ones. This manner of dying, which was imposed by panicked public health measures, and then exploited by newspapers, was perhaps the biggest tragedy of all. Treating infection towards the end of a life-limiting illness rather than providing palliation, makes the dying process that much harder, but this is what we witnessed during COVID-19. How much of what we experienced have we understood?

Rather than oxygen and ventilators, well known and effective palliative care measures could have reduced the shortness of breath symptoms as well as the anxiety that often accompanies the sensation of asphyxia in the dying. Analgesics such as morphine have been frequently used with great success in those dying from other types of terminal lung conditions such as pulmonary fibrosis or COPD. Such treatments in a palliative care setting for those dying from COVID-19 were then, and are now, preferable to invasive life-saving measures that did not work and were never desired. Were such palliative care measures taken for those afflicted with COVID-19 in Nursing Homes as they died? This may be a hard but necessary question to ask if we are to learn something from this pandemic.

If, before the pandemic broke out, more people had a Palliative Care or an Advanced Care Plan in place that did not include resuscitation, potentially thousands of families could have chosen to continue looking after their ailing loved-ones with COVID-19 *at home*, under voluntary quarantine if needed. They could have chosen to do so with or without personal protective equipment (PPE), instead of enduring a painful and often harmful separation due to a hospitalization that often included unwanted technological support. Knowing their loved one's end-of-life wishes in advance, or even their own wishes for their loved one, would have given caregivers the option for them to close the eyes of their loved one, instead of an unknown "staff" person, a recurring theme also reported in print and electronic news media, further augmenting the fear and the panic.

According to the Oxford definition, panic is "sudden, uncontrollable fear or anxiety, often causing wildly unthinking behaviour." We saw this spread with lightning speed through our various media channels, leading to a global phenomenon of unprecedented restrictions and lock down measures. In this type of environment, supporting quality of life and a dignified, peaceful death which most of our ailing seniors desired, did not stand a chance. Instead, thanks to the media frenzy, whole societies got swept away by alarm. Our knee-jerk desparation to "conquer the virus" brought the battlefield to the very people who wanted to die peacefully rather than "take up arms."

Sadly, our governments, our media, our medical organizations, and our societies failed these people. We failed because we forgot that death is part of life. We failed because we forgot that for most people, but especially for the elderly, quality of life far outweighs in importance length of life. We failed because we panicked. When we put these people into our frightened shoes, instead of slipping into theirs, we acted without thinking. Trying to save their lives at any cost, brought upon them and their families a most undeserved, terrible, and irreversible harm. This, and not their deaths, is the real tragedy.

In our current fallen state, where we await the resurrection of the dead and the Second Coming of our Lord God and Savior Jesus Christ, death is part of life. We expect people living in nursing homes or with a life-limiting illness to eventually die.[25] It is normal at all times, not just pandemic times, for the oldest, weakest, and most ailing members of society to succumb to death more easily than those who are younger, stronger, and healthier. The role of society in general and the medical profession in particular is not to prevent death at any cost, but to support both the living and the dying as they wish to be supported, with dignity. This is the essence of person-centred care and equitable access, which we should aspire to and maintain at the forefront of all medical care in any circumstance—especially, the circumstance of a pandemic such as COVID-19.

Now that we have all intimately experienced our first global pandemic in one way or another, perhaps we have learned something new. I hope we have learned that our future pandemic planning should include affording people the option to die from it at home, in the presence of their loved ones, with appropriate palliative care supports. I hope we have learned how important it is to ensure that everyone, but especially those with at least one life-limiting illness, prepare an Advanced Care Plan (that includes a pandemic plan) before the next pandemic strikes. We should think

---

25. During the first wave of the Covid-19 pandemic, 81% of Canadian COVID-19-associated deaths occurred in nursing homes where the majority of residents have at least one life-limiting illness. See Globe and Mail: https://www.theglobeandmail.com/canada/article-new-data-show-canada-ranks-among-worlds-worst-for-ltc-deaths/.

about providing PPE to caregivers in the home, if they wish it, as we do to hospital and nursing home staff.

If we do this, instead of repeating the tragic headlines of 2020, the number of people and their families who choose a home death in the next pandemic may surprise us. It may even surprise us if the next pandemic does not fill up our hospitals, or cause a panic!

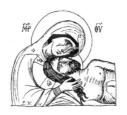

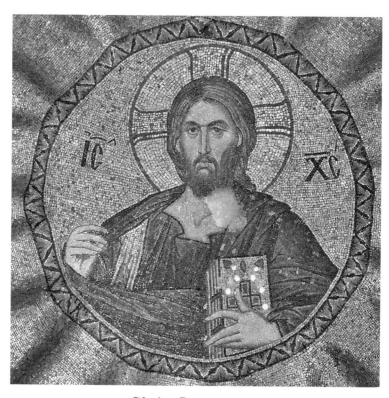

Christ Pantocrator

CHAPTER 6

In Whom Do You Put Your Trust? An Orthodox Analysis of COVID Science

Deacon Ananias Erik Sorem, Ph.D.

An unanticipated consequence of the COVID-19 crisis since early 2020 is the ways by which and through which "science" has vaulted to the forefront of public concerns and conversations. Since everyone presupposes something about science and has various precommitments in forming beliefs, approaching factual questions, observing evidence, etc., our first task in this chapter will be to identify and 'quarantine,' as it were, the corrupted science and "scientism" promoted by the technological, medical, pharmaceutical, and political elites that are fueling the COVID-19 phenomenon. Then we shall explore how "good" science can undergird an authentic, realistic, and proper response to the coronavirus disease and its proposed remedies from an Orthodox Christian perspective.

The Philosophical Challenge

Whether one takes a realist, a critical realist, an instrumentalist, or a metaphysical quietist philosophical position on science,[1] what becomes evident from the literature and history is that science does not reach the level of knowledge that the average layman and those who ascribe to "scientism" think it does. This has particular significance for our considerations of the COVID science, since most who support the official stance on COVID, together with their prescribed recommendations, ascribe a greater epistemic status to science than it really has. One of the issues that plague our common and contemporary views of science (a factor that often leads to scientism) is a fundamental confusion between methodology (methods for obtaining desired results) and ontology (reality). Because of the pragmatic success of the methodology in modern science, many of us are led to think that science gives us an exalted, objective, or comprehensive knowledge of the world.

However, the pragmatics of methodology do not necessarily equate to knowledge of reality (i.e., just because it works does not mean that it is true). For example, the Quine/Duhem underdetermination of data thesis[2] allows for multiple conflicting scientific paradigms and theories whose individual methodologies all "work" and whose descriptions all fit the appearances/data, but nevertheless cannot all be "true," because they contradict one another. Michael Polanyi has observed that the "premises of science

---

1. These are various positions taken within the philosophy of science concerning what science describes, its goals, what we can know, and what—if anything—exists.

2. The Quine-Duhem Theory of the Underdeterrmination of Data thesis shows that our data, sense-experience, and observations can all fit and support multiple conflicting scientific theories or paradigms: i.e., the available evidence at any given time will be insufficient for determining what theory or beliefs we should adopt. Therefore, what passes for "science" exceeds the limits of the evidence / data.

on which all scientific teaching and research rest are the beliefs held by scientists on the general nature of things."[3] Anthony O'Hear is more direct: "Much of what scientists tell us of these things inevitably goes way beyond anything we have evidence for. Any evidence we have is necessarily drawn from a tiny part of the whole universe and may not be representative or indicative of the whole."[4] Taking this in conjunction with how science has currently been elevated to the status of absolute truth,[5] we have reason to suspect that what is presented as COVID science may be corrupted by "scientism." Therefore, let us turn our attention to this issue.

The Gnosticism of Scientism

Systems have arisen in history where science ceased being science, yet nevertheless, operated under the guise of science. In this instance, the imposter of science, scientism, is a modern type of gnostic heresy[6] that claims to have, if not the fullness

---

3. Michael Polanyi, *Science, Faith, and Society* (Chicago: Chicago University Press, 1946), 11.

4. O'Hear, *An Introduction to the Philosophy of Science*, (Oxford: Oxford University Press, 1989), 203.

5. As O'Hear states, "the elevation of fascinating speculation into absolute truth is one of the marks of a mythology." Ibid., 204.

6. Voegelin lists six characteristics of gnosticism: "(1) It must first be pointed out that the gnostic is dissatisfied with his situation. This, in itself, is not especially surprising. We all have cause to be not completely satisfied with one aspect or another of the situation in which we find ourselves. (2) Not quite so understandable is the second aspect of the gnostic attitude: the belief that the drawbacks of the situation can be attributed to the fact that the world in intrinsically poorly organized. For it is likewise possible to assume that the order of being as it is give to us men (wherever its origin is to be sought) is good and that it is we human beings who inadequate. But gnostics are not inclined to discover that human beings in general and they themselves in particular are inadequate. If in a given situation something is not as

of truth, at least more truth than the original prototype. Eric Voegelin identifies both Marxism and National Socialism, although not limited to them, as examples. In such socio-political structures, the society at large and most scientists in those societies remove God as the intelligible ground of being, that which would ground science, and they begin to create speculative enterprises and systems that make certain questions both practically and conceptually impossible.[7]

For example, for Karl Marx his concealment in his gnostic speculation takes the form of an "intellectual swindle." Voegelin states:

> Marx's prohibition of questions has to be characterized as an attempt to protect the 'intellectual swindle' of his speculation from exposure by reason; but from the standpoint of the adept Marx the swindle was

---

it should be, then the fault is to be found in the wickedness of the world. (3) The third characteristic is the belief that salvation from the evil of the world is possible. (4) From this follows the belief that the order of being will have to be changed in an historical process. From a wretched world a good one must evolve historically. This assumption is not altogether self-evident, because the Christian solution might also be considered – namely, that the world throughout history will remain as it is and that man's salvational fulfillment is brought about through grace in death. (5) With this fifth point we come to the gnostic trait in the narrower sense – the belief that a change in the order of being lie in the realm of human action, that this salvational act is possible through man's own effort. (6) If it is possible, however, so to work a structural change in the given order of being that we can be satisfied with it as a perfect one, then it becomes the task of the gnostic to seek out the prescription for such a change. Knowledge—gnosis of the method of altering being is the central concern of the gnostic. As the sixth feature of the gnostic attitude, therefore, we recognize the construction of the formula for self and world salvation, as well as the gnostic's readiness to come forward as a prophet who will proclaim his knowledge about the salvation of mankind" (Eric Voegelin, Science, Politics, and Gnosticism, 64-65).

7. "The murder of God, then, is of the very essence of the gnostic re-creation of the order of being." (Eric Voegelin, *Science, Politics, and Gnosticism*, 41)

the 'truth' that he had created through his speculation, and the prohibition of questions was designed to defend the truth of the system against the unreason of men.[8]

Questions about what constitutes genuine science are also suppressed. Other conceptually impossible actions within the neo-gnostic systems include the questioning of the "settled science." When anyone proffers an alternative, that explanation garners yet another speculative explanation that can be neither verified nor falsified. Hence, the "science" that is incapable of falsification moves out of the realm of science and into the domain of pseudo-science. Voegelin goes on to argue that this takes on a religious quality and becomes known as scientism instead of science.

Augusto Del Noce points out that "the distinctive ideology of the 'technological society' is scientism, the 'view of science' as the 'only' true knowledge..." This, he argues inevitably leads to a technocratic totalitarianism: "Now, an advocate of scientism, and a society based on his way of thinking, cannot help being totalitarian inasmuch as his conception of science . . . cannot be the object of any proof . . . but does not intend to elevate other forms of thought to a higher level . . ., he simply 'denies them.'"[9] Scientism not only employs non-falsifiable methods, but the totalitarian tactic of social feeling (social group think, which can be enforced through media, education, politics, corporations, the state, etc.) is used to enforce the "settled science." The positivist founders of scientism, Saint-Simon and Comte, advocated for the

---

8. Eric Voegelin, Science, Politics, and Gnosticism, (Wilmington, DE: ISI Books, 1968), 11.

9. Augusto Del Noce, *The Crisis of Modernity*, (Montreal: McGill-Queen's University Press, 2015), 231.

use of "social feeling" tactics to subordinate individuals and conform them ideologically to the new system in the name of "progress." Voegelin identifies these things as essential components of gnostic systems and key features of scientism.

There is a definite link between scientism and technocracy. Neil Postman states:

> By Scientism, I mean three interrelated ideas that, taken together, stand as one of the pillars of Technopoly . . . [1] the methods of the natural sciences can be applied to the study of human behavior . . . [2] social science generates specific principles which can be used to organize society on a rational and humane basis. This implies that technical means—mostly "invisible technologies" supervised by experts—can be designed to control human behavior and set it on the proper course . . . [3] faith in science can serve as a comprehensive belief system that gives meaning to life, as well as a sense of well-being, mortality, and even immortality.[10]

What should concern us is that we have encountered these elements—attitudes, thought processes, technological possibilities, and human behaviors—since the emergence of the "COVID science." In fact, it is something that existed prior to the COVID-19 virus in the "settled science" of Evolutionary Theory, and more recently, climate change. Many scientists believe as truth the Theory of Evolution, despite its unalterable failure to satisfy the Scientific Method—the very definition of science. This is a classic example of "settling the science" in the absence of true

---

10. Neil Postman, *Technopoly*, (New York: Vintage Books, 1993), 391.

science. Although there may be scientists who believe in God, a large majority of scientists and the social and political system that supports scientific research operate on secular atheistic assumptions. This current system is historically situated in our post-Enlightenment, technocratic-gnostic socio-political structure. Furthermore, as the philosopher of science, Anthony O'Hear, points out, "If science itself can take on some of the characteristics of mythology, it is also true that science, being part of culture produced by human beings, cannot remain immune from other cultural and ideological influences"[11] and inevitably will be shaped by technocratic ideas and powers. Therefore, let us look at various epistemological techniques to determine the trustworthiness of certain scientific claims and see how certain ideologies and the power structure may corrupt science and medicine.

Epistemic Litmus Tests for Good Science.

Philosophers often propose thought experiments and scenarios that, although we may never encounter them in real life, serve as epistemic tools to derive certain principles, confirm or falsify various theories, test hypotheses, etc. For example, we need only to think of Descartes' evil demon thought experiment to illustrate that it did not reveal that he believed everything was an illusion and deception created by an evil demon but was an attempt to show that under the worst-case scenario some things could or could not be known with certainty. Taking this in conjunction with something like Popper's falsification principle (the attempt

---

11. Anthony O'Hear, *An Introduction to the Philosophy of Science*, 210.

to disprove one's theory, rather than confirm it), we may find a helpful heurism in establishing whether we can trust the COVID science presented to us. Let us assume the worst-case scenario for which, I shall argue below, there is evidence and see if the prevailing narrative concerning the COVID science is trustworthy.

Consider the following epistemic litmus test in the form of a question to determine how we would know whether something is good or bad science. What special methodology, unique insight, or appeal to distinct privileged paradigms would you, as an individual scientist, use that would allow you to know that what passed for actual science (in Hitler's Nazi dictatorship, Stalin's Communist Russia, or any Marxist regime) was genuine science instead of science corrupted by dominant ideologies or propaganda? What would make you personally and uniquely distinct from all the rest of the people or scientists in those regimes, when a substantial majority agreed the science was settled, true, authoritative, and provided justification for carrying out certain extreme measures in the name of the "common good"? Now ask yourself, how do you know that you are not in a similar situation now? How could you know? Will the science reveal that to you, or will those individuals who represent the science and who provide or communicate the "official scientific stance reveal that to you?" Once the official scientific stance is revealed, then what would constitute evidence that the "official scientific stance" is trustworthy, presupposing that real or true evidence should not merely consist of a confirmation given by certain chosen "experts." The epistemic litmus test for good science (real evidence / truth) occurs when questions are freely permitted to create a healthy introspection, active investigation, and fair and open debate. That is necessary for a person to exercise independent free will and apply reason, judgment, and factual evidence, rather than a facile acceptance or blind faith in authority.

In our present predicament we can use similar techniques employed by detectives and prosecutors to determine the trustworthiness of a person or a group, applying these techniques to the current COVID-19 narratives to determine whether "the science" is operating properly as science should. Let us call these techniques "detective epistemology," but, before we examine them, let us turn our attention to the topic of technocracy.

What is Technocracy?

Broadly defined, technocracy is the governing or control of society by an elite group of technical experts – but what is technocracy precisely, how did it originate, and how is it relevant to us? The seeds of technocracy begin in earnest with Saint-Simon and Auguste Comte's positivism and their scientism, following a radical shift in thinking about technology and the meaning of knowledge during the "scientific revolution" in the 17th century and the Enlightenment in the 18th century. For example, it was Francis Bacon who famously declared that "Human knowledge and human power is the same thing, for where the cause is not known the effect cannot be produced."[12] Not only is knowledge redefined purely in terms of pragmatic and predictive effects,[13] a new science, a new morality, new aesthetics, and a new philosophy are created—in short, a new world. As Phillip Sherrard notes,

---

12. Francis Bacon, *Novum Organum* (Englewood Cliffs, NJ: Prentice Hall), 3.

13. Comte offered this famous dictum: *Savoir pour prevoir* ("To know in order to predict").

When Bacon concluded that his novum organum should apply 'not only to natural but to all sciences' (including ethics and politics) and that it is to 'embrace everything,' he opened the road for the all-inclusive scientific takeover of our culture and for the urban industrialism which is its brainchild.[14]

This is the Baconian prescription for "the total scientization of our world . . ."[15] In his New Atlantis, Bacon "conceived of a new social order dedicated to the expansion of modern science and progress in human achievement through dominion over nature . . . "[16] Modern mechanization was perfected in the likes of Galileo, Descartes, and Newton, whose projects accept only a universal quantitative approach to everything and the application of mathematical techniques to all of nature. In this new social order, anything that does not submit to this universal quantitative project simply is not science. As Sherrard explains, "what could not be caught in the net of numbers was non-science, non-knowledge, and even in the end non-existent."[17] This, together with the revolutionary spirit[18] of the new man, who in his self-

---

14. Phillip Sherrard, "Modern Science and Dehumanization," *Studies in Comparative Religion*, Vol. 10, No. 2. (Spring, 1976), 8.

15. Ibid.

16. John G. Gunnell, "The Technocratic Image and the Theory of Technocracy," *Technology and Culture*, Vol. 23, No. 3 (July 1982), 394.

17. Phillip Sherrard, "Modern Science and Dehumanization," 8.

18. "For modern science has its starting-point in a revolution in consciousness, or revolt against heaven, that has resulted in the reason first ignoring, then denying, and finally closing itself to the source of knowledge which is above it; and this has meant that it has been forced to turn for its knowledge exclusively to that which is below it—to the "external" world of sense-data and sense-impression." Ibid., 13.

proclaimed autonomy revolted against heaven, resulted in a period that "is characterized by the increasing dominance of anthropocentric forms of political speculation, as opposed to theocentric questions."[19] Mircea Eliade, a scholar of world religions, defined modern societies as "those which have pushed the secularization of life and the Cosmos far enough."[20]

According to the precepts of modernity, as typified by the Enlightenment thinking of Kant, not only must we conceive of nature and her laws as radically autonomous and independent of God, the Promethean rebellion against God must also apply to the human will. Both nature and the human will, are now considered radically autonomous from God. An autonomous mechanized nature and humanity leaves us without any objective meaning or grounding in the transcendent. As Bruce Foltz concludes, "such a world offers no inner resistance to manipulation and control, presents no grain against which we ought not to cut. In Heidegger's words, it is a world that has become an inventory or resource (in German, *Bestand*) for technological control and consumption."[21] Technology, therefore, is now promoted as the sole means to exploit nature to and recreate man and society according to the gnostic and atheistic insistence to

---

19. Dante Germino, *Machiavelli to Marx: Modern Western Political Thought*, (Chicago: University of Chicago Press, 1972), 7.

20. Mircea Eliade, *Myths, Dreams, and Mysteries: The Encounter Between Contemporary Faiths and Archaic Realities* (New York, NY: Harper and Row, 1975), 25.

21. Bruce Seraphim Foltz, "The Gnosticism of Modernity and the Quest for Radical Autonomy," (Paper presented at *Orthodox Anthropology and Secular Culture in the 21st Century Conference*, Holy Trinity Orthodox Seminary, Jordanville, NY, March 7-9, 2019), 3.

perfect the human experience without grounding it in the living God as the unconditioned grounds of being.[22]

How does this concept of technology relate to the idea of technocracy? The political power of the secular state, which attempts to maintain a canonical morality over a relativistic and nihilistic culture that embraces a plurality of moralities,[23] has been exchanged for a "New Atlantis." Political institutions, as John Gunnell points out, have begun to be "replaced by a 'parliament' of technical experts."[24] This elite class of technical experts are now technocrats. The technocratic image[25] now replaces the politician and provides mankind with a "vision of an industrial society wherein an elite class of engineers, scientists, industrialists, and planners systematically apply technical knowledge to the solution of social problems and the creation of a rational social order."[26]

---

22. The late Orthodox bioethicist Tristram Engelhardt saw morality grounded "not in philosophy but in an experience of the living God who commands."—H. Tristram Engelhardt Jr., *After God: Morality and Bioethics in a Secular Age*, (New York: St. Vladimir's Seminary Press, 2017), 217.

23. "After metaphysics and after God, the secular fundamentalist state becomes a surrogate for God because, once reality, morality, and bioethics are severed from an unconditioned ground in being, and once moral reason is recognized as plural in content, one is not just left with a plurality of moralities and bioethics, but also the closest thing to a common morality and a common bioethics becomes that morality and bioethics are established as law and in public policy . . ." (Engelhardt, After God, 92-93).

24. John G. Gunnell, "The Technocratic Image and the Theory of Technocracy," 394.

25. "Many of the characteristic features of the technocratic image may be found in the work of Henri de Saint-Simon (1760-1825) and his vision of an industrial society wherein an elite class of engineers, scientists, industrialists, and planners systematically apply technical knowledge to the solution of social problems and the creation of a rational social order" (John G. Gunnell, "The Technocratic Image and the Theory of Technocracy," 394).

26. John G. Gunnell, "The Technocratic Image and the Theory of Technocracy," 396.

Many of their ideas and social engineering techniques ("social physics") undergird our current "science." These prominent intellectuals in the 20th century articulated the technocratic theory and ideology: Max Weber, Karl Mannheim, Edward Bellamy, Bertrand Russell, Arthur Koestler, Zbigniew Brzezinski, et. al.

The term "technocracy" originated with an engineer in 1919 named William Smith and achieved familiarity as an idea in response to the Great Depression in the 1930s. John Gunnell explains that technocracy as an ideology "for a time gained considerable notoriety and a substantial following," and

> began with a group of technicians and engineers dedicated to social reform whose concepts were modeled on the technological republic in Edward Bellamy's late-19th-century utopian novel Looking Backward. They were also influenced by the economic theories of Thorstein Veblen and the principles of scientific management growing out of the work of Frederick W. Taylor, both of which suggested, much like the later work of James Burnham in The Managerial Society, that politicians and industrial entrepreneurs should, and would, give way to technical elites.[27]

C. P. Snow, who dramatically pursued the problem of the influence of experts on political decisions, argued that "one of the most bizarre features of any advanced industrial society in our time is that the cardinal choices have to be

---

27. John G. Gunnell, "The Technocratic Image and the Theory of Technocracy," 393.

made by a handful of men" in a world of "closed politics" and "secret scientific choices" where there is "no appeal to a larger assembly . . . in the sense of a group of opinion, or electorate."[28]

Technocracy is intrinsic to the socio-political system and policymaking in a unique way. John Gunnell explains technocracy's relation to politics as follows:

1. In circumstances in which political decisions necessarily involve specialized knowledge and the exercise of technical skills, political power tends to gravitate toward technological elites.

2. Technology has become autonomous; hence politics has become a function of systemic structural determinants over which it has little or no control.

3. Technology (and science) constitute a new legitimating ideology that subtly masks certain forms of social domination.[29]

Again, much of this goes back to Saint-Simon and Comte's positivism. Concerning Saint-Simon, Dante Germino explains that there was "a mania for system construction characteristic of the nineteenth century in particular . . . He was obsessed with the urge to reduce all explanations, all principles to a single over-arching formula. There could be only one science, one government, one religion, one organization of social classes."[30] Saint-Simon's

---

28. C.P. Snow, Science and Government (Cambridge, MA: Harvard University Press, 1961), 1.

29. John Gunnell, "The Technocratic Image and the Theory of Technocracy," 397.

30. Dante Germino, *Machiavelli to Marx*, 280.

progressivism, socialism,[31] and positivism would all coalesce into the ideology of scientism, providing the technological managerial ruling elite of the future technocracy with their own religion.[32] In keeping with one of H.G. Wells' predictions, the technological elite can use religion for social domination to control populations and the socio-political structures.[33] The underlying condition that allows a technocracy to arise and corrupt science, control policy making, manipulate research, and result in certain forms of social domination is the scientism that arises from modernity. However, before getting into how technocracy specifically ties into the current science concerning COVID, let us return to our epistemological discussion about evidence, trust, and justification.

Establishing Trustworthiness

The 1976 swine flu that infected 230 soldiers at Fort Dix, New Jersey, and resulted in one death led to the "fast tracked" production of a vaccine and instructions to all Americans from the corporate-medical establishment and the U.S. government, to get vaccinated. After forty-five million Americans were vaccinated, four thousand Americans filed vaccine damage claims with the federal government totaling

---

31. "Saint-Simonians were among the first to use the term 'socialism,' which entered the Western political vocabulary in the late 1820s" (Ibid, 283).

32. "Scientists began to take the place of priests, initiating not of course into the kingdom of heaven but into the brave new world of more consumer goods and limitless economic growth. It was by courtesy of the scientists that the industrialists and bankers of the nineteenth century bulldozed their way to fortune and produced the devastation of the modern industrial world" (Phillip Sherrard, "Modern Science and Dehumanization"), 8.

33. See H.G. Wells' *God the Invisible King*

$3.2 billion. Three hundred deaths were attributed to the vaccine, together with several hundred cases of Guillain-Barre syndrome, which led to paraplegia in some healthy young adults.

Something similar occurred with the H5N1 bird flu scare of 2005, when President Bush had declared that two million people would die from the bird flu.[34] However, despite all the fear and hysteria, only 98 persons died globally in 2005 and another 115 the following year, hardly a pandemic.[35] What resulted were fast-track procedures for licensing and approval of pandemic vaccines created by the World Health Organization (WHO): "Ways were sought to shorten the time between the emergence of a pandemic virus and the availability of safe and effective vaccines."[36] This should sound familiar.

Then, there was the unwarranted swine flu scare of 2009 and warnings that it could kill 90,000 Americans and hospitalize two million human beings. These numbers were never actualized, but the Centers for Disease Control (CDC) pushed for universal immunization with Swine Flu vaccine, despite the moderate severity of the Swine Flu, which did not typically require hospitalization. We see similar patterns today with the COVID-19 pandemic.

---

34. George W. Bush, "National Strategy for Pandemic Influenza: Implementation Plan," Published May 2006. https://georgewbush-whitehouse.archives.gov/homeland/pandemic-influenza-implementation.html.

35. "In 2005, 98 people died globally, and another 115 the following year." Jeffrey Tucker, "A Retrospective on the Avian Flu Scare of 2005," *American Institute for Economic Research*, Published online March 22, 2020. www.aier.org/article/a-retrospective-on-the-avian-flu-scare-of-2005/.

36. World Health Organization, "Safety of Pandemic Vaccines: Pandemic (H1N1) 2009 Briefing Note 6," Published August 6, 2009, https://www.who.int/csr/disease/swineflu/notes/h1n1_safety_vaccines_20090805/en/.

Despite the similarities, there is a striking socio-political difference between previous outbreaks and the Covid-19 pandemic. The Swine Flu of 1976, which resulted in vaccine related deaths and injuries, also led to $3.2 billion of damage claims with the American federal government. Prior to the Covid-19 vaccine rollout, governments absolved manufacturers of any liability related to vaccine injury or death. This did not pose a major problem while immunization was voluntary. When the following year, in 2021, these same vaccines were unexpectedly mandated in many sectors, a historical precedent of forced individual choice was set, between a vaccine and job loss, with no legal recourse for vaccine injury and no pharmaceutical accountability – hardly a just or democratic circumstance for first world countries.

The legal question *"Cui bono?"* (Who benefits?) applies here. In each viral outbreak since 1976, we have seen the same pattern of behavior —a rapidly derived vaccine that is endorsed as the only solution. This benefits Big Pharma and Big Tech (essential parts of the technocracy), providing a motive for inflated numbers of cases and deaths. The latter in turn creates more fear, excessive governmental control, and the suppression or censoring of other evidence that would question or contradict the meme of "pandemic," or point to safer, or more effective, or less expensive treatments, other than the novel and expensive vaccines that Big Pharma has prescribed and marketed. That American COVID-19 deaths are exaggerated, has been confirmed by The John Hopkins University, supporting a repeat of the same pattern of mass hysteria followed by mass vaccination evident in previous flu outbreaks.[37]

---

37. Yanni Gu, "John Hopkins University Reveals Manipulated Covid Death

Let us now examine the relation between drug companies and the American medical community to understand the level of corruption between scientific research and the practice of medicine.

Drug Companies and Doctors as a Source of Corruption

The cronyism among drug companies (Big Pharma), the medical and research establishments, and government is a major source of corruption that often prevents, or at least interferes with, the conduct of good science and the practice of good medicine in the USA, and, by extension, quite possibly in other countries.

Dr. Marcia Angell, MD, former Editor in Chief of the *New England Journal of Medicine* (a prestigious and leading medical journal) published an article in January 2009 titled, "Drug Companies and Doctors: A Story of Corruption,"[38] which examines how corporate-academic liaisons have corrupted the integrity of medicine. As mentioned earlier, pharmaceutical companies are highly motivated to exaggerate diseases, promulgate fears, and promote (by misinforming and even lying) about their drugs to benefit financially from their sales.[39] Since drug companies provide

---

Figures," *Sign of the Times*, Published online November 22, 2020. www.sott.net/article/444898-Johns-Hopkins-University-Reveals-Manipulated-Covid-Death-Figures.

38. Dr. Marcia Angell, MD, "Drug Companies and Doctors: A Story of Corruption," *The New York Review*, Published online January 15, 2009, http://www.nybooks.com/articles/22237.

39. "To promote new or exaggerated conditions, companies give diseases or bodily afflictions serious-sounding names along with abbreviations. Thus, heartburn is now 'gastro-esophageal reflux disease' or GERD; impotence is 'erectile dysfunction' or ED; premenstrual tension is 'premenstrual dysphoric disorder'

major funding for research, Dr. Angell argues that they can easily introduce bias and corrupt the integrity of medicine and science:

> Because drug companies insist as a condition of providing funding that they be intimately involved in all aspects of the research they sponsor, they can easily introduce bias to make their drugs look better and safer than they are. Before the 1980s, they gave faculty investigators total responsibility for the conduct of the work, but now company employees or their agents often design the studies, perform the analysis, draft the papers, and decide whether and in what form to publish the results.[40]

This results, Dr. Angell argues, in scientists and medical faculty becoming "little more than hired hands, supplying patients and collecting data according to instructions from the company."[41]

---

or PMMD; and shyness is 'social anxiety disorder' (no abbreviation yet). Note that these are ill-defined chronic conditions that affect normal people, so the market is huge and easily expanded. For example, a senior marketing executive advised sales representatives how to expand the use of Neurontin: 'Neurontin for pain, Neurontin for monotherapy, Neurontin for bipolar, Neurontin for everything.' It seems that the strategy of the drug marketers—and it has been remarkably successful—is to convince Americans that there are only two kinds of people: those with medical conditions that require drug treatment and those who don't know it yet. While the strategy originated in the industry, it could not be implemented without the complicity of the medical profession" (Dr. Marcia Angell, "Drug Companies and Doctors: A Story of Corruption").

40. Ibid.

41. Ibid.

That, in turn, leads to manufactured control and conflicts of interest that lead to further problems in the scientific and medical communities.

Since 2020, we have already seen a strong correlation between the push for the mRNA vaccines and the suppression of alternative medicines and treatments for the corona virus. According to Dr. Angell, the "industry-sponsored trials published in medical journals consistently favor sponsors' drugs, largely because negative results are not published, positive results are repeatedly published in slightly different forms, and a positive spin is put on even negative results."[42] Dr. Angell also points out that, in psychiatry alone, a

> review of seventy-four clinical trials of antidepressants, for example, found that thirty-seven of thirty-eight positive studies were published. But of the thirty-six negative studies, thirty-three were either not published or published in a form that conveyed a positive outcome. It is not unusual for a published paper to shift the focus from the drug's intended effect to a secondary effect that seems more favorable.[43]

This type of maneuvering inevitably leads to physicians practicing "a very drug-intensive style of medicine. Even when changes in lifestyle would be more effective, doctors and their patients often believe that for every ailment and discontent there is a drug."[44]

---

42. Ibid.

43. Ibid.

44. Ibid.

A similar type of manipulation surrounds the management of COVID-19, where reasonable and possibly good alternatives to technologically novel and potentially harmful vaccines are suppressed.[45] Furthermore, many physicians are either forced or choose to believe that the newest technology is superior to anything else, despite any risks, since many doctors are both funded (which we will discuss in further detail) by these drug companies and are also "swayed by prestigious medical school faculty, to learn to prescribe [these] drugs... without good evidence of effectiveness." *The Lancet* (a highly respected peer-reviewed medical journal) exposes pharmaceutical misinformation from drug companies, by discussing the true efficacy of the mRNA COVID-19 vaccines. While Pfizer and Moderna claim a 95% and 94% efficacy relatively speaking, these values represent the relative risk reduction (RRR) rather than the more accurate and much lower absolute risk reduction (ARR), to give the appearance that the vaccines are more effective than they actually are.[46] The clearest way to inform a true understanding of the efficacy of a product is with the Number Needed to Treat (NNT) which is 119 for Pfizer's and 81 for Moderna's mRNA vaccines. The NNT is the

---

45. See Dr. Robert Malone's (inventor of the mRNA technology) interview with Bret Weinstein, "How to Save the World in Three Easy Steps," Dark Horse Podcast on Odyssey, Published online June 18, 2021, https://podcasts.apple.com/us/podcast/how-to-save-the-world-in-three-easy-steps/id1471581521?i=1000525032595 and Steve Kirsch's research on the dangerous of the mRNA vaccines and evidence of more effective alternative treatments in his article "Should you get Vaccinated," TrialSite News, Published online May 25, 2021, https://trialsitenews.com/should-you-get-vaccinated/.

46. Lancet Microbe. "COVID-19 Vaccine Efficacy and Effectiveness—the Elephant (not) in the Room," Published online April 20, 2021, www.thelancet.com/journals/lanmic/article/PIIS2666-5247(21)00069-0/fulltext

number of people who need to receive the vaccine to prevent one case of illness. Neither Pfizer nor Moderna legally lied, because the RRR *is* a type of efficacy, but the RRR value does not mean what most doctors and non-physicians alike think it means. This tactic is used by the majority of pharmaceutical companies to impress potential buyers and users and is highly effective in securing the acceptance and the sale of a product. From the the user's or recipient's perspective, believing in (trusting) the science, or scientism, reduces skepticism and facilitates unquestioning acceptance.

Dr. Angell also explains the corruption that arises from the funding of doctors by drug companies in the United States this way: "[M]ost doctors take money or gifts from drug companies in one way or another. . . No one knows the total amount provided by drug companies to physicians, but I estimate from the annual reports of the top nine US drug companies that it comes to tens of billions of dollars a year."[47] She concludes that the pharmaceutical industry through funding has "gained enormous control over how doctors evaluate and use *its* own products. Its extensive ties to physicians, particularly senior faculty at prestigious medical schools, affect the results of research, the way medicine is practiced, and even the definition of what constitutes

---

47. "Many are paid consultants, speakers at company-sponsored meetings, ghost-authors of papers written by drug companies or their agents, and ostensible 'researchers' whose contribution often consists merely of putting their patients on a drug and transmitting some token information to the company. Still more doctors are recipients of free meals and other out-and-out gifts. In addition, drug companies subsidize most meetings of professional organizations and most of the continuing medical education needed by doctors to maintain their state licenses" (Dr. Marcia Angell, "Drug Companies and Doctors: A Story of Corruption").

a disease."[48] The biases and conflicts of interest and that result in corrupted science and medicine are not restricted to psychiatry, and the sources of corruption are not limited to drug companies: "Similar conflicts of interest and biases exist in virtually every field of medicine, particularly those that rely heavily on drugs or devices."[49] Consequently, as Dr. Angell explains, "It is simply no longer possible to believe much of the clinical research that is published, or to rely on the judgment of trusted physicians or authoritative medical guidelines."[50] Substantially drastic measures require substantial evidence, which having considered just a few of the aforementioned points, is far from being sufficient for such drastic measures. Furthermore, "drug companies have perfected a new and highly effective method to expand their markets . . . ," where instead "of promoting drugs to treat diseases, they have begun to promote diseases to fit their drugs . . . ," a strategy "to convince as many people as possible (along with their doctors, of course) that they have medical conditions that require long-term drug treatment . . . "[51] Based on this information, we have ample reason to think that the science and data regarding COVID-19 have been manipulated in favor of financially benefiting the pharmaceutical industry.

In addition to this type of unreliability in scientific and medical circles, there are countless published research studies of low quality science. In 2015, Richard Horton, editor of The Lancet, wrote, "Much of the scientific literature, perhaps

---

48. Ibid.
49. Ibid.
50. Ibid.
51. Ibid.

half, may simply be untrue. Afflicted by studies with small sample sizes, tiny effects, invalid exploratory analyses, and flagrant conflicts of interest, together with an obsession for pursuing fashionable trends of dubious importance, science has taken a turn towards darkness."[52] Dr. John Ioannidis, one of the world's leading experts in medical research at Stanford University, adds that 90% of medical research is tainted and flawed due to influence from the pharmaceutical industry.[53] This gives greater cause for concern that a degree of corruption has played a role in the COVID-19 vaccine rollout.

The role of drug companies in technocracy and their cronyism with other entities further compounds the problem of corruption in science and medicine. As the tendency for political power to gravitate toward technological elites such that science and technology become autonomous, the technocracy makes politics a function of systemic structural determinants, over which politicians have no control. We can see how the collusion among various institutions, including Big Tech, Big Pharma, the medical establishment, regulating bodies, universities, corporations, financial institutions, foundations, the mainstream media, the entertainment and music industries, nation-states, and various transnational players, generates similar global and local solutions to the

---

52. Dr. Richard Horton, "Offline: What is medicine's 5 sigma?", *The Lancet*, Vol. 385, Published online April 11, 2015, www.thelancet.com/journals/lancet/article/PIIS0140-6736(15)60696-1/fulltext.

53. Dr. Ioannis tells David H. Freedman in his article, "Lies, Damned Lies, and Medical Science," that as much as 90 percent of the published medical information that doctors rely on is flawed." (Freedman, "Lies, Damned Lies, and Medical Science," *The Atlantic*, Published November 2010. www.theatlantic.com/magazine/archive/2010/11/lies-damned-lies-and-medical-science/308269/.)

social, economic, ecological, and health issues related to COVID-19. However, any global effort on a global issue or concern is bound to be toothless without the cooperation of national governments and their ability to act and legislate to support their aims. Nation-states make global governance possible (one leads the other), which is why the United Nations Organization insists that "effective global governance can only be achieved with effective international cooperation."[54] Klaus Schwab maintains that the "two notions of global governance and international cooperation are so intertwined that it is nigh on impossible for global governance to flourish in a divided world that is retrenching and fragmenting."[55]

Thus far, we understand that science does not exist in a vacuum. As we have seen, science is embedded within certain socio-political structures and operates on the assumptions of those dominating ideologies.[56] Therefore, our current science ought to be assessed in light of the current gnostic technocracy and its philosophy (scientism and the technocratic image of man and the future society), an overall ideology that results in control, conflicts of interest, biases, the favoring of sponsors' drugs and research, the suppression of contrary or negative evidence, and various other perversions that permeate the

---

54. United Nations, Department of Economic and Social Affairs (DESA), Committee for Development Policy, "Global governance and global rules for development in the post-2015 era," Policy Note, 2014, Accessed June 3, 2021, www.un.org/development/desa/dpad/wp-content/uploads/sites.

55. Klaus Schwab, *COVID-19: The Great Reset*, (Geneva, Switzerland: Forum Publishing, 2020), 82.

56. "Specific Authority demands therefore not only devotion to the tenets of a tradition but subordination of everyone's ultimate judgment to discretionary decision by an official center." Michael Polanyi, Science, Faith, and Society. (Chicago: The University of Chicago Press), 59.

scientific and medical fields.[57]   Again, scientific analysis at this paradigm level will inevitably involve epistemological questions concerning recent problems beseting nutrition science, climate change, and COVID science that raise issues of trust.

Considering the current gnostic technocratic totalitarian system and cronyism outlined above, we find that many of our current problems are not due to random errors, insufficient sample sizes, or invalid exploratory analyses. A "specific authority" can indeed corrupt the scientific judgments and procedures[58] of the dominant gnostic technocratic system by determining the main scientific narrative and promulgating its ideas through the structures and institutions already mentioned, that are managed and controlled by the technocratic elite. Of course, "social feeling," as Saint-Simon and Comte point out, also becomes necessary to control and determine people's thoughts and actions ("manufactured consent," according to Noam

---

57. "In view of this control and the conflicts of interest that permeate the enterprise, it is not surprising that industry-sponsored trials published in medical journals consistently favor sponsors' drugs. Negative results are ignored, while positive results are published repeatedly in slightly different forms, and negative results receive a positive spin. A review of seventy-four clinical trials of antidepressants, for example, found that thirty-seven of thirty-eight positive studies were published. [Erick H. Turner et al., "Selective Publication of Antidepressant Trials and Its Influence on Apparent Efficacy," *The New England Journal of Medicine*, January 17, 2008.] But of the thirty-six negative studies, thirty-three were either not published or published in a form that conveyed a positive outcome. It is not unusual for a published paper to shift the focus from the drug's intended effect to a secondary effect that seems more favorable" (Dr. Marcia Angell, NY Review of Books, January 15, 2009, "Drug Companies & Doctors: A Story of Corruption").

58. See Michael Polanyi, Science, Faith and Society. (Chicago: The University of Chicago Press, 1946).

Chomsky).[59] This gnostic concealment tactic of "social feeling" is fully on display in recent attempts to shut down questions concerning many things: whether the COVID-19 data collected is accurate, whether the tests are reliable, whether the available treatments are sufficiently effective, safe or ethical, whether the mandates, the restrictions and other measures are justifiable, whether fear-mongering, injustice or corruption has been used to manipulate the population, etc.. We often receive pseudo-scientific "non falsifiable" responses to many of these questions such as, "It didn't work because we didn't lock down long enough," or "Not enough people were wearing masks," when none of these measures was rigorously studied in the first place to demonstrate any degree of efficacy. This is another indicator that the supposed "science" is no longer science, an essential sign of a modern gnostic system in Voegelin's terms. To be sure, that does not mean good science does not exist, but it does illustrate how non-science can masquerade as "science."

Let us now return to the techniques employed by detectives and prosecutors to determine the trustworthiness of the official COVID-19 pandemic story, by considering some of the "court room type" evidence surrounding human behavior, prior criminality, motive, and other factors. If the **behavior** of a suspect includes intimidation of witnesses, concealing or destroying evidence, arbitrary censoring, demonetizing, de-platforming, accusing critics of "conspiracy theories," or changing his or her story (narrative) or alibi, then that suspect's name climbs higher on the list of suspects as either "guilty," or protecting a guilty party. A **history**

59. See Edward Herman and Noam Chomsky's book, Manufacturing Consent (New York: Pantheon Books, 1988).

of corruption, lying and manipulating data, as in the case of Pfizer,[60] makes repeated corruption more plausible. Financial gain also provides a strong motive. If a pandemic preparation plan provides detailed and accurate predictions of how our current pandemic has played out vis a vis the social, political and media responses,[61] it can be held akin to reading a detailed fictional murder story, only to discover afterwards that such a murder actually took place. Would such a finding not make the author of the story more suspect as the murderer? Considering all this evidence, together with the fact that (1) several prominent newspapers, magazines, and major media corporations are funded by the same foundations,[62] and (2) various trans-national players all share a common ideology and goals and benefit financially from their cooperation,[63] and (3) the underlying commitment to

---

60. Although there have been other cases, the most notable case of pharmaceutical fraud was announced by the Department of Justice on September 9, 2009 when they published that Pfizer was found criminally and civilly responsible for illegally promoting certain pharmaceutical products, submitting false claims about their products to government and health care programs, and paying kickbacks to health care providers to induce them to prescribe these drugs. This resulted in the largest health care fraud settlement in history. www.justice.gov/opa/pr/justice-department-announces-largest-health-care-fraud-settlement-its-history.

61. See, for example, the exercise known as Event 201, the John Hopkins Center for Health Security document, *The SPARS Pandemic 2025—2028*, Accessed May 31, 2021, www.auricmedia.net/wp-content/uploads/2020/12/spars-pandemic-scenario.pdf.

62. For example, among the various Gates Foundation grants, $250 million has gone to the following major media corporations, all of which have routinely published news favorable to Gates and his projects: BBC, NBC, Al Jazeera, ProPublica, National Journal, The Guardian, Univision, Medium, The Financial Times, The Atlantic, The Texas Tribune, Gannett, The Washington Monthly, Le Monde, PBS NewsHour, and the Center for Investigative Reporting.

63. For further information on shared goals and partnerships, see the World Economic Forum and their list of partners, www.weforum.org/partners/. Also see the World Health Orgnization and their partnerships, www.healthcluster.who.int/

scientism is precisely what makes it possible to "manufacture consent" and corrupt the science,[64] we have more than enough reasons to doubt the "official narrative" concerning COVID-19 and substantial evidence of social engineering and manufactured consent.

How Did We Get Here?

We can trace the problem at hand back to a fundamental shift in thinking and orientation that occurred in modernity. Modern man began to view himself, the world, the cosmos, the polis, and his proper place in relation to them all in a radically different way from the ancients. In his Promethean rebellion, man severed the transcendent ground of being, from the intelligible world and declared a self-proclaimed autonomy whereby he believed he could exercise full dominion over being (the world and the entire cosmos). In his Nietzschean deicide, modern man created speculative gnostic systems, and, like Adam and Eve, he attempted to hide his sin by using his system to conceal the truth. Man's abolition of both the transcendent God and nature resulted in a loss of objectivity, something that would have restrained his immoral thoughts, and actions. Consequently, the libido dominandi became the only guiding principle, a sheer will to power where man could use (or misuse) technology to control,

---

partners. Shared goals among transnational actors and instutions can be found documented in the United Nations, Department of Economic and Social Affairs (DESA), Committee for Development Policy, "Global governance and global rules for development in the post-2015 era", Policy Note, 2014, www.un.org/en/development/desa/policy/cdp/cdp_publications/2014cdppolicynote.pdf.

64. See Edward Herman and Noam Chomsky's book, Manufacturing Consent (New York: Pantheon Books, 1988).

dominate, and exploit nature in the name of "science" and progress.

For the modern man, "the speculative system in which the gnostic unfolds his will to make himself master of being" demands to be called "science."[65] However, to commit such deeds, science had to become absolutized and, with it, the entire world scientized—the very essence of Scientism. It "is, literally, a resolution of the will: the resolution to accept as real only what can be verified empirically by everyone."[66] Nevertheless, to effect a complete scientization of the world, Scientism had to relate to the socio-political sphere. Hence, the atheistic gnostic speculators created what is known as technocracy. Within our current technocratic totalitarian system, we have found another gnostic ideology that is dehumanizing, anti-scientific, atheistic, and completely at odds with Christianity. Since such gnostic systems corrupt science, we must be aware of their presence, dominion, and power to corrupt. Furthermore, we must acknowledge that technocratic totalitarianism, like all modern gnostic systems, attempts to conceal these sins by building a socio-political operating system that prevents asking foundational paradigmatic questions, making such questions practically and conceptually impossible.

Where do we go from Here?

What, then, is the solution to our current gnostic scientism and technocratic totalitarianism, beyond just becoming

---

65. Eric Voegelin, Science, Politics, and Gnosticism (Wilmington, DE: ISI Books, 2004), 32.

66. Augusto Del Noce, The Age of Secularization (Montreal: McGill-Queen's University Press, 2017), 104.

aware of it? As Sherrard himself explains, "It is superfluous to stress that this cosmic disorder, reflecting the radical dehumanization of our society, incurable apart from a total re-personalization of the conditions of work in our society, is already well advanced . . . " Since "our society cannot be re-personalized or rehumanized without a dismantling of the whole present scientific industrial structure, we have something of the measure of the task that lies ahead."[67] If, however, we are to rebuild our "society in the image of an integrated humanity, we must first be clear in our minds what it means to be human."[68] Since the idea of what it means to be human in Christianity is not the same as in the secular atheistic technocracy of Scientism, we must first admit that there is simply no common ground here.[69]

This is something of which Tristram Engelhardt himself was keenly aware, particularly in the domains of bioethics and medical science. There is no common ground with secularism because, as Engelhardt argues, the secularists' "goal is to have secular professional ethics trump other moral obligations, including one's obligations to God. 'Selfless' secular professionalism and social justice are thus invoked as objective moral norms that require health professionals to violate their 'private' obligations to God . . . "[70] He

---

67. Sherrard, "Modern Science and Dehumanization," 5.

68. Ibid.

69. In fact, as Carlo Lancellotti in his article "Augusto Del Noce on the 'New Totalitarianism'" states: "the technological society is no longer unified by any shared idea of the good..." ("Augusto Del Noce on the 'New Totalitarianism.'" *Communio* 44, Summer 2017 (Communio: International Catholic Review), 326), and, therefore, there cannot be a common ground with a society that does not have any unified, shared idea of the good, let alone an idea of the Christian good.

70. H. Tristram Engelhardt, *After God*, 254.

warns us that secularism means that our Christian paradigm and "commitment to honor one's obligations to God is characterized as a self-centered, selfish focus on private matters or private religious 'feelings' that are inferior in their force and that conflict with, and are overridden by, public secular social obligations . . . "[71]

Therefore, given the preponderance of evidence concerning the conflicts of interest within the industry and the power structures and financial incentives of the groups identified as the technocracy, who are not only capable of corrupting the science for financial gain and ideological control, but have a known history of such crimes, why would one trust the "official narrative" concerning COVID-19? What would one's evidence be that such a system is trustworthy—evidence that would not be anecdotal or result in question begging, such as citing doctors or scientists who support one side but are precisely those who are questionable themselves? Again, why would the various explanations supporting the "official narrative" not be equivalent to a non-falsifiable conspiracy theory?

These questions are the most important questions to ask, especially since our most credentialed and experienced living holy elders, ascetics, and monks (who have removed themselves from secular ideological influences) speak with one voice[72] against the "official COVID-19 narrative" and its prescriptions. Meanwhile, those of us "in the world," as we say, including priests and bishops, who are most susceptible

---

71. Ibid.

72. Speaking with "one voice" is meant to suggest that there is a clear consensus among our holy elders, monks, and ascetics. It does not mean that everyone holds the exact same position within that community concerning this issue.

to influences from secular ideas and politics, compromised in numerous ways, and / or misled by other distractions, are divided on this issue. We Orthodox Christians conduct our epistemology by looking for consensus, especially among the credentialed spiritual elders, where the highest epistemological status is attained through a life of repentance and asceticism (the places where monks living apart from "the world" spend most their time), and not through placing the primacy on philosophy and science to achieve these epistemological heights. Therefore, we Orthodox need to acknowledge that the true consensus stands firmly against the "official COVID-19 narrative" and its prescriptions. In other words, it is the Orthodox practice of repentance and asceticism that illumines our philosophy and science, and not the other way around. Each Orthodox Christian must look within and ask, "In whom do I put my trust?"

Here we find two worlds beckoning to us: a city of man and a city of God. We are reminded of the Gospel passage that warns us "No one can serve two masters. Either you will hate the one and love the other, or you will be devoted to the one and despise the other."[73] Pluralism and multiculturalism are failed experiments. Secular pluralistic societies attempt to blend contradictory cultures, values, and ideologies. However, since the core values, morals, ideas, and commitments of distinct cultures and competing philosophical systems are fundamentally at odds with one another, it is inevitable that one group will have to compromise its essential beliefs. This creates a situation where the will of the stronger alone resolves ideological conflicts, an appeal once again to the gnostic principle of libido dominandi. In our current crisis,

---

73. Matthew 6:24

it is the atheistic technocratic totalitarians, using the secular state under the spell of "science" who exercise their will to overpower and eliminate any competing ideologies or practices. Multicultural and pluralistic anthems are simply Trojan horses, bringing in an enemy whose ideas and ethos are irreconcilable with Christianity. As Engelhardt observes, "We do not share common ground. Christianity has ancient roots that are immune from the consequences of the collapse of the Western moral-philosophic project."[74]

The two paradigms, the Christian and the modern secularist, represent conflicting worldviews that are simply incompatible with one another. Within law, government, education, ethics, science, medicine, and society at large, we find ideological conflicts, as well as conflicting prescriptions for a person's conduct in each of these venues. We continue to confront claims about science and what constitutes proper medical care that are simply at odds with Christianity. We need only consider the numerous bioethical conflicts to acknowledge "the incompatibility of claims made by the contemporary secular state about what should count as proper medical professional conduct and those claims grounded in the demands of God."[75] Moreover, the public policy and health guidelines regarding COVID-19 that the secular state and technocratic elites champion and strive to enforce often contradict our liturgical practices and faith. We have identified several problems with the absolutizing of science, which precludes critical assessments of the latest scientific claims and approaches. We have highlighted the dangers of Scientism and pseudo-science, as well as pointing

---

74. Tristram Engelhardt, *After God*, 389.

75. Ibid., 19.

out general concerns about trusting a science that is now operating within the framework of a gnostic atheistic and antihuman technocracy.

The real krisis (judgment) for us is how we shall judge and decide. Where and in whom do we put our trust? Do we put our trust in the city of man or the city of God? Do we put our trust in the secular, immoral, anti-Christian technocrats (where "science," I have argued, no longer operates as science), elevating the empirical sciences (the lowest form of reasoning) with its ever-changing conclusions to the status of divine revelation and absolute truth? Or do we put our faith in the lives of the Saints, the life of the Church, in the Faith once delivered to us by God Himself, the Faith of the Orthodox, the Faith that established the Universe? It is not clear how Christians in the present crisis can help to fashion a suitable environment to conduct science and politics. However, it is my hope that through this crisis we begin to see the religious nature of the threat at hand. It is my hope that we can identify the corruption of philosophy into philodoxy that culminates in the radical transformation of the political / social framework that would otherwise make science intelligible. As I have argued, we now exist in a new social-political-paradigmatic order, where science has become a religion of its own and an enemy of true religion. The new religion is Scientism or science-idolatry, where the high priests are the scientific "experts"[76] and technocratic

---

76. "Scientists began to take the place of priests, initiating not of course into the kingdom of heaven but into the brave new world of more consumer goods and limitless economic growth. It was by courtesy of the scientists that the industrialists and bankers of the nineteenth century bulldozed their way to fortune and produced the devastation of the modern industrial world" (Sherrard, "Modern Science and Dehumanization," 8).

elites, and the devotees and worshipers are those who participate in the gnostic structures of the totalitarian terror of technocracy. As Voegelin reminds us,

> Today, under the pressure of totalitarian terror, we are perhaps inclined to think primarily of the physical forms of opposition. But they are not the most successful. The opposition becomes radical and dangerous only when philosophical questioning is itself called into question, when doxa ["glory"] takes on the appearance of philosophy, when it arrogates to itself the name of science and prohibits science as nonscience.[77]

We have entered a new age based on the old reoccurring gnostic themes. We find an absolutizing of science (replacing philosophy, epistemology, ontology, and metaphysics with empirical sciences), an elevation of the "technical experts" to the infallible magisterium of the new universal religion, and the suppression—if not complete abolition—of all questioning and critical analysis of their project and their new gnostic religion. There has, as Voegelin explains, "emerged a phenomenon unknown to antiquity that permeates our modern societies so completely that its ubiquity scarcely leaves us any room to see it at all: the prohibition of questioning."[78] Although these modern gnostic projects and speculative programs (as opposed to philosophy) have existed in the political paradigms of socialism, Marxism, and National Socialism, the "conscious, deliberate, and painstakingly

---

77. Eric Voegelin, *Science, Politics, and Gnosticism*, 15.

78. Ibid., 16.

elaborate obstruction"[79] of logos has not been limited to these paradigms. We are living in the gnostic scientism of the technocratic totalitarianism of this present age.

We ought to count this as a blessing. For a crisis will make things clearer to us. It will help us see to what ideas, beliefs, and values we are committed. It will aid us in seeing where we put our faith and trust. Let us not forget, as the Optima Fathers in Russia pray: "Teach us to treat that whatever may happen with peace of soul and with firm conviction that Your will governs all . . . . In unforeseen events, let us not forget that all are sent by you."[80] This crisis is the will of the Lord. Glory to God! Let us make the best of it and ask ourselves whom do we serve and where is our citizenship? Let us say, as the people said to Joshua, "I will serve the Lord." With the grace and help of God, let us resist the spirit of the age and this world and declare, as the Psalmist says, "Some trust in chariots and some in horses, but we trust in the name of the LORD our God."[81]

May we pray that, on that dreadful judgment day, our Lord and Savior, Jesus Christ will say to us "well done good and faithful servant"[82] and not "I never knew you; depart from Me."[83]

---

79. Ibid.

80. Prayer of the Optina Fathers," *Orthodox Prayer Book* (Lake George, CO: New Varatic Publishing, 1990), 13.

81. Psalm 20:7 KJV

82. Matthew 25:23

83. Matthew 7:23

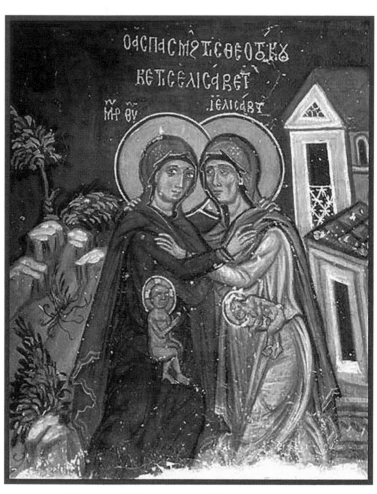

Prenatal Forerunner Prostrating to
Prenatal Christ

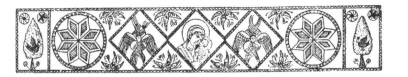

CHAPTER 7

The Moral Peril of Taking Most COVID-19 Vaccines[1]

Archpriest Alexander F. C. Webster, PhD

The familiar epigram "sometimes the cure is worse than the disease" applies perforce to the COVID-19 crisis since the advent of the current vaccines. The worldwide Orthodox Church is riven on the morality of those vaccines. Fully acknowledging the tragic number of deaths and debilitating physical harm to many of the survivors of this virus, I shall argue in this chapter that an unanticipated "side effect" of receiving the vaccines currently available is, from an Orthodox Christian moral perspective, a *post-factum* collusion in the original intrinsically evil acts of abortion that enabled those vaccines to be produced and/or tested and made available around the world.

---

1. This chapter is a substantial revision, expansion, and updating of a previous version that appeared under the same title on the monomakhos.com Orthodox blog on April 15, 2021. I am grateful to George Michalopoulos and Gail Shepherd for including the earlier version on their website.

I. Advocates of the Vaccines

A. Hierarchs and Synods

Let us consider first prominent Orthodox hierarchs who make a case in favor of any of the COVID-19 vaccines currently available in their respective nations.

An online article on January 16, 2021, reported that "Metropolitan Hierotheos of Nafpaktos and Agios Vlasios became" in December 2020 "one of the first people to receive one of the vaccines in Greece. The occasion was filmed, and he said people would enjoy higher life expectancy thanks to the vaccine." The entire Holy Synod of Greece also announced in mid-January 2021 that they would defer to "science," since the vaccines currently in use in Greece did not require "embryonic cell cultures for their production."[2] For the Synod that meant the following: "The Holy Synod reiterates that the choice of vaccination is not a theological or ecclesiastical issue. It is mainly a medical-scientific issue, as well as a free personal choice of each person in communication with his doctor, (sic) and does not constitute a fall from the right faith and life."[3]

Six months later in July 2021 the Standing Holy Synod sent an encyclical to all the dioceses of the Orthodox Church of Greece titled, "Church and Science in the Fight Against the Pandemic." That document declared:

---

2. "Orthodox Church undermines Greece's COVID pandemic measures": https://www.dw.com/en/orthodox-church-undermines-greeces-covid-pandemic-measures/a-56251674 (Accessed on December 15, 2021)

3. Holy Synod quoted in ibid.

[T]oday, the Church trusts the scientific community of doctors, which fights day and night for the liberation of people from the deadly pandemic.

In fact, it is emphasized that humanity now has at its disposal the vaccine, "which is capable of building a wall in the spread of the pandemic. The Standing Holy Synod of the Church of Greece, knowing that vaccination is a maximum act of responsibility towards fellow humans, recommends to everyone, in consultation with their doctor, to use the gift that God has given us, to protect ourselves, and others.

The Church of Greece genuinely wants to assure that this vaccine does not come in any contradiction with the Hagiographic, Patriarchal and Canonical teaching of our Holy Church."[4]

The Holy Synod of Greece at that time also encouraged the faithful to take the COVID-19 vaccine as "the exclusive and scientifically tested solution to stop the virus."[5] It is quite clear that the Orthodox Church in Greece is committed body (medically) and soul (Church teaching) to the various COVID-19 vaccines. I shall argue below that the hierarchs of that esteemed autocephalous Church are incorrect in

---

4. Quoted in "Church of Greece: The vaccine does not contradict the teaching of our Holy Church," *Orthodox Times*, July 20, 2021: https://orthodoxtimes.com/church-of-greece-the-vaccine-does-not-contradict-the-teaching-of-our-holy-church/ (Accessed on December 15, 2021).

5. "Church of Greece: Vaccination is the Only Solution to Stop the Virus," https://orthodoxtimes.com/church-of-greece-vaccination-is-the-only-solution-to-stop-the-virus/ (Accessed December 15, 2021)

their hasty moral assessment of the vaccines. The Synod's understanding of the "science" in this case is also lacking. It is true that aborted preborn baby cells *per se* are not integral components of most COVID-19 vaccines. However, each of the vaccines currently available relies on aborted preborn baby cell lines derived from aborted baby organs that served as the original source for multiple laboratory processes that resulted in a final product—a "cell line"—on which each of the current COVID-19 vaccines was derived, or tested, or both. A direct connection to the original aborted preborn baby cell is, therefore, both undeniable and morally culpable, protests to the contrary notwithstanding.

Playing bad cop to Metropolitan Hierotheos' good cop, Metropolitan Chrysostomos of Dodoni in Greece has decided to compel the faithful to receive a COVID-19 vaccine. On a local radio program on July 14, 2021, he announced this alarming decision:

> I called a deacon with my successor, asked him and he told me he had not been vaccinated. I told him, until you think about getting a vaccine, going home, you have no right to come with people. If grandparents are forced to be vaccinated, it will be an example for the rest of those who are not vaccinated. Believers are influenced by some priests or some fools. The metropolitans should put them on holiday. 'Vaccination must be mandatory for everyone who is not at home and for every employee who is in the public sector.'[6]

---

6. "Palavous" characterized the thousands of Greeks who demonstrated by Metropolitan Dodonis: "Let's vaccinate them compulsorily" (Accessed on July 16, 2021): https://www-pronews-gr.translate.goog/thriskeia/1002141_palavoys-harak-

Raising the ante in the COVID-19 stakes in the Greek-speaking world, Archbishop Chrysostomos II of the ancient autocephalous Orthodox Church of Cyprus, said to the Omega television channel viewers in Cyprus:

> Today, I made an announcement to the Archdiocese; when they get back to work because in a week we go on vacation, those who have not been vaccinated must be vaccinated. Those who are not vaccinated should not go back to work.
>
> They must consider themselves fired; I will fire them and I do not discuss this with anyone. They are either persuaded and get vaccinated or they are fired. That is all.
>
> They should learn to respect others. I will convene the Holy Synod very soon after the holidays because everyone has to come down to earth.[7]

In an interview in Kyiv, Ukraine, on August 20, 2021, no less an esteemed leader than the Patriarch Bartholomeos of Constantinople (in Istanbul, Turkey), traditionally the most senior of the heads of autocephalous Orthodox Churches around the world, offered a bold endorsement of the COVID-19 vaccines, while caricaturing the objections of others to the vaccine and shaming them in print, and

---

tirise-toys-hiliades-ellines-poy-diadilosan-o-mitropolitis-dodonis?_x_tr_sl=auto&_x_tr_tl=en&_x_tr_hl=en&_x_tr_pto=ajax,elem (Accessed on December 15, 2021).

7. "Archbishop of Cyprus: The Archdiocese Employees Who are Not Vaccinated Will be Dismissed," *Orthodox Times*, July 20, 2021: https://orthodoxtimes.com/archbishop-of-cyprus-the-archdiocese-employees-who-are-not-vaccinated-will-be-dismissed/ (Accessed on December 15, 2021).

revealing that he and the other leaders at the patriarchal headquarters had taken one of the vaccines:

"[T]he refusal of vaccination and other protection measures is irrational and unjustified by theological or scientific criteria. I have said from the beginning that the pandemic threatens our faithful, but not our faith. It is true that a large number of believers who refuse protection measures are victims of this virus. That is why it is unacceptable to deny the existence of a pandemic, to regard it as created by someone, or to spread conspiracy theories in the face of so many victims and so much suffering. Unfortunately, this attitude shows indifference to others. However, anything that contradicts the commandment to love one's neighbor cannot be the will of God. The Church of Constantinople urges the faithful to consult with their doctors and to vaccinate according to their instructions. Naturally, all of us at Fanari, including me, were vaccinated."[8]

Meanwhile in the United States, the Assembly of Canonical Orthodox Bishops of the USA (or AOB) issued on January 22, 2021, a "Statement Regarding Developments in Medicine: COVID-19 Vaccines & Immunizations." The hierarchs, representing nine Orthodox jurisdictions,[9] made the same case as the Holy Synod of the Church of Greece

---

8. The interview was reported in *UKRINFORM*, "the only national news agency of Ukraine": https://www.ukrinform.ua/rubric-society/3301395-jo-go-vsesvatist-varfolomij-arhiepiskop-konstantinopola-novogo-rima-i-vsel-enskij-patriarh.html?fbclid=IwAR36xYOTGm27OlxNTCS2y2X4iNu2u71J-yp_W6CkbnTiccgnDqY2ZEoGZbIQ

9. Not including its erstwhile member, the Russian Orthodox Church Outside Russia, which withdrew from the AOB on October 15, 2018, pursuant to a eucharistic schism between the mother Church in Russia and the Patriarchate of Constantinople over the latter's uncanonical intervention in a decades old ecclesial dispute in Ukraine.

for an odd—and disturbing—separation between medical and spiritual realms when they declared:

> We therefore encourage all of you—the clergy and lay faithful of our Church—to consult your physicians in order to determine the appropriate course of action for you, just as you do for surgeries, medications, and vaccinations, in cancer treatments and other ailments. Indeed, while your own bishop, priest, or spiritual father remains prepared to assist you with spiritual matters, your personal doctor will guide your individual medical decisions.
>
> We trust that whatever course of action you and your doctor decide upon will also benefit the rest of the community.[10]

What may appear in that Statement as prudent respect for the "medical" sciences is instead, I contend, an abandonment of the fullness of "spiritual" truth revealed in the Orthodox moral tradition, which we dare not quarantine and render irrelevant to our personal decisions about bodily health.[11]

---

10. https://www.assemblyofbishops.org/assets/files/messages/AoB%20Exec%20Co%20Medicine%20Statement.pdf (Accessed on December 16, 2021).

11. Ironically, in stark contrast to those canonical Orthodox bishops, The North American Diocese of The Russian Orthodox Church Abroad (ROCA), a schismatic entity recognized by neither the canonical Russian Orthodox Church Outside Russia (ROCOR) nor the mother church, the Patriarchate of Moscow, has issued a strong statement against the COVID-19 vaccines: "The Russian Orthodox Church Abroad does not bless its members to accept any of the COVID vaccines. These are not traditional vaccines, but a program designed to override and manipulate the natural immune system of the body. These vaccines are only experimental and stand to do irreparable harm to a person's [sic] God given immune system. In addition, they contain and/or use aborted human infant tissue in their production [sic]. Consequently, the Church cannot and will not bless anyone to accept these vaccines and strenuously warns everyone against accepting them."

Archbishop Elpidophoros and the Holy Synod of the Greek Orthodox Archdiocese of America, which always chairs the Assembly of Bishops in the USA, taking a cue from a similar decision by the New York archdiocese of the Roman Catholic communion in America communicated to its priests on July 30, 2021,[12] announced the following six weeks later, on September 16, 2021:

> Discussing the topic of the vaccination of the faithful, the hierarchs unanimously affirmed that the Church not only permits vaccinations against diseases (e.g., polio, smallpox), but that She encourages Her Faithful, after medical tests and approbations, to be vaccinated with the approved vaccines against SARS-CoV-2 (COVID-19).
>
> In addition, although some may be exempt from the vaccination for clear medical reasons, there is no exemption in the Orthodox Church for Her faithful from any vaccination for religious reasons, including the coronavirus vaccine. For this reason, letters of exemption for the vaccination against the coronavirus for religious purposes issued by priests of the Archdiocese of America have no validity, and furthermore, no clergy are to issue such religious exemption letters for any reason.
>
> The Holy Eparchial Synod urges the faithful to pay heed to competent medical authorities, and to avoid the false narratives utterly unfounded in science

See http://rocana.org/archives/14332 (Accessed on December 16, 2021).

12. https://www.americamagazine.org/faith/2021/08/03/religious-exemptions-covid-vaccine-catholic-241167 (Accessed on December 16, 2021).

and perpetrated on the Church by those who have succumbed to the disinformation and conspiracy theories that are widely available on social media sites.[13]

That *a priori* suppression of dissenting Greek Orthodox clergy is alarming, because it takes the crisis to a new level of authoritarianism by preempting all theological reflection, discussion, and action on the subject. It also bodes ill for other Orthodox jurisdictions that may be tempted to join ranks with the Greek Archdiocese and suppress their clergy. Meanwhile, what does the GOA now have to offer faithful, conscientious Orthodox laity whose careers, jobs, military service, or college education may hinge on a letter of support from a priest for their religious exemption from the COVID-19 vaccines?

Meanwhile, in Russia at least three widely respected bishops have resorted to extreme rhetoric or drastic decisions in favor of the Sputnik V vaccine, which, like all the others currently available, has a direct link to an aborted preborn baby cell-line.

In June 2021, Metropolitan Hilarion (Alfeyev) of Volokolamsk, head of the Department for External Church Relations of the Russian Orthodox Church, expressed a "'positive attitude' towards the government initiative to impose compulsory vaccination on those working in the service sector."[14] In an interview with a Russian television

---

13. "Communique of the Holy Eparchial Synod," September 16, 2021: http://byztex.blogspot.com/2021/09/greek-archdiocese-dissolves-all.html (Accessed on December 16, 2021).

14. "Refusing to be vaccinated against Covid-19 is a 'sin' & anti-vaxxers must spend their life repenting, says Russian Orthodox Church": https://www.rt.com/russia/528425-orthodox-church-anti-vaxx-sin/ (Accessed on December 16, 2021).

news station on July 5, 2012, the Metropolitan intensified his public position. Conceding that "it is desirable to observe the principle of voluntariness (sic) in relation to vaccinations—the principle that was stated from the very beginning," he reminded the faithful nonetheless that "there is also the principle of people's responsibility for the lives of other people." Referring to Orthodox faithful who had refused to take the vaccine and felt guilty for passing the COVID 19 virus to someone who subsequently died from the disease, Metropolitan Hilarion offered this startling, unpastoral message during his interview: "They come and say, 'How am I supposed to live with this now?' And it's hard for even me to say how to live with it. . . . All your life, you have to make up for the sin you committed."[15]

A few weeks later in another interview with RT TV in Russia, Metropolitan Hilarion (Alfeyev) doubled down on his firm position albeit without the invocation of sin:

> I am told: why do you so actively call people to be vaccinated? Indeed, you have no medical education. And one does not have to be a medic to see what is happening around, in what agony people with the coronavirus die. They simply suffocate. It is a nightmarish death. Such patients cannot even say goodbye to their relatives, as the latter are not allowed to see them. Doctors see all that; we, priests, see that. Compared to what is happening, the anti-vaccination rhetoric seems simply absurd and even sacrilegious. That is why I am not shy of speaking, in both my programs and other public appearances: God has

---

15. Ibid.

sent to us now an opportunity for getting rid of the coronavirus pandemic, so let us use this opportunity.

Parishioners often ask me: when will all this come to an end? When this pandemic began, we did not know when it will come to an end because we did not have an 'antidote.' Now we have it—there are three Russian vaccines. If you do not like one, take another.[16]

The French website Orthodixie.com published an article on July 12, 2021, that provided an imbedded video in which Metropolitan Tikhon (Shevkunov) addressed the Russian Orthodox faithful of the Archdiocese of Pskov.[17]   He revealed that he had already received a COVID-19 vaccine three times!

[A]t the end of August [2020] I was vaccinated against covid with Sputnik-V. The vaccination went perfectly, I noticed nothing. . . . But in April, my antibody level dropped so much that I was advised to get the vaccine again, and just recently, ten days ago, the doctors advised me to get the vaccine for the third time. They explained to me that the current Indian strain of the virus is very aggressive, and able to overcome even a medium level of good immunity. Only high immunity is able to protect a person from this disease. And the second and third time I had no

16. "Metropolitan Hilarion: Through common efforts we will manage to overcome the pandemic": https://mospat.ru/en/news/87694/ (Accessed on December 16, 2021).

17. Jivko Panev, "About vaccination, emergency appeal from Metropolitan Tikhon (Shevkunov)," July 12, 2021: https://orthodoxie.com/a-propos-de-la-vaccination-appel-durgence-du-metropolite-tikhon-chevkounov/ (Accessed on December 16, 2021).

side effects. And I know a lot of people who have not only been vaccinated but revaccinated with different vaccines.

A strong advocate for the Sputnik V vaccine and yet opposed to mandatory vaccination of his flock, Metropolitan Tikhon shockingly threatened resistant priests and monks in his jurisdiction with unspecified canonical penalties if anyone whom they dissuaded from the vaccine were to suffer serious illness or death:

> As the Bishop of the Pskov Diocese, who is responsible for the flock entrusted to me by God, of course, I give my unconditional blessing to take into account all the recommendations of the Russian State Health Service and to carry out preventive vaccinations against this deadly disease that is covid. I take this responsibility, I make this recommendation, and of course I respond. Of course, I am responsible to my herd. And I think it's fair. The time for empty words is over.
>
> But at the same time, I must say that those priests (there are few in our diocese, but they do exist) who divert their flock and their friends from preventive vaccinations should also be held responsible. It is clear that this is their opinion. They think it's the right thing to do. But if—God forbid—anyone among those who did not get the vaccine because you dissuaded them from getting it becomes seriously ill or dies (and in the hospital, you will certainly know that they were not vaccinated precisely because this or that priest did not bless them to do so—the person who will be sick will explain to the doctor the reason for his actions), if, God

forbid, this happens, then these priests or monks will have to endure full canonical responsibility for these acts.

But even that guilt-tripping of his clergy was not the most outrageous action of a hierarch in Russia. On June 24, 2021, the RIA-Novosti news service in Moscow quoted Bishop Pankraty of Troitsk, abbot of the renowned Valaam Monastery on an island in the Karelia region of Russia, who contracted COVID-19 in September 2020 *after* receiving the Sputnik V vaccine:

> I stand for absolutely complete, one hundred percent vaccination of the entire population of the Russian Federation. This is my position: I was just myself in the red zone, dying, I saw people waiting to die on mechanical ventilation, the question is—when will they die? (sic) who came in a grave condition. Therefore, some polemics, some opinions, they are absolutely inappropriate.

Any of the two hundred monks and employees at Valaam who refuse to take the vaccine, Bishop Pankraty declared, "are simply removed from the monastery without any maintenance."

However, RIA-Novosti reported that pilgrims who visit the monastery "will be asked by the monastery to provide certificates of vaccination or results of PCR tests. Bishop Pankraty added, 'But if we are vaccinated, then we will not be so scared.'"[18]

---

18. "On Valaam, residents who have not been vaccinated will be expelled from the monastery": https://ria.ru/20210624/valam-1738507428.html (click

After howls of protest both within Russia and around the world over the prospect of casting skeptical monks out of the monastery with no means of support, the Russian Orthodox Church mercifully overruled the Valaam abbot. Bishop Savva of Zelenograd, Deputy Administrator of the Moscow Patriarchate, announced in a Russian "Telegram" tweet on July 1, 2012, "As for Valaam, as of today, there is no more talk of compulsion. Vladyka Pankraty is trying to exhort the brethren in a fatherly way. There can be no question of 'eviction' due to non-vaccination."[19]

B. Professor Tristram H. Engelhardt's Nuanced Argument

A sophisticated, nuanced ethical argument in favor of all COVID-19 vaccines currently available and in production, though one that, in my estimation, ultimately fails to reflect Orthodox moral tradition in its fullness, appears in chapter 5 of the late Tristram H. Engelhardt's book, *Foundations of Christian Bioethics* published in 2000.[20] In that chapter the distinguished professor takes square aim at what he terms

---

on "English"; Accessed on July 15, 2021).

19. "No Mandatory Vaccination at Valaam, Says ROC Deputy Administrator": https://orthochristian.com/140251.html (Accessed on December 16, 2021). The same article also reported this news item: "President Vladimir Putin stated that he is against mandatory vaccination and explained that State Duma Deputies also opposed making the COVID vaccine mandatory on the federal level. However, according to a 1998 law, regional leaders have the right to introduce mandatory vaccination for certain categories of citizens on the recommendation of their local chief sanitary doctor."

20. Tristram H. Engelhardt, *Foundations of Christian Bioethics* (Beverly, MA: Scrivener Publishing, 2000).

the "Emerging Secular Liberal Cosmopolitan Consensus" in bioethics.[21]

Early in that chapter, Engelhardt condemns unequivocally what traditional Orthodox moral theologians term the intrinsic evil of all abortions even in so-called hard cases: "The taking of human life, even the life of unborn children in order to preserve the life of the mother, always falls short of the pursuit of holiness: *abortion is always wrong* [NOTE: italics added]. Persons are not just those who can now act as moral agents, but all who are called to worship God eternally."[22] He also presents what any traditional Orthodox Christian would deem sound bioethics on a host of other pressing contemporary questions. "Surrogate motherhood," he observes, "even if undertaken in order to rescue an unborn child, would still involve a significant dissociation of reproduction from the unity of marriage. Though the acceptance of zygotes for surrogate gestation could be interpreted as the saving of early human life, one must avoid immoral actions, even if these will save the life of others."[23] One would expect, therefore, a similarly high moral standard and cogent argument when he addresses the question of the "use of tissues and organs from fetuses (sic) who have been aborted."[24] But that is where Engelhardt's bioethics goes off the rails.

Alas, Engelhardt presents a clear argument for the morality of vaccines connected to aborted preborn baby cell-lines in this short section on p. 261 (boldface added for emphasis):

---

21. Ibid.
22. Ibid. 238.
23. Ibid. 257.
24. Ibid. 261.

Under circumstances that allow the use of tissues and organs from persons who die accidentally, it is **appropriate to use tissues and organs from fetuses who die accidentally**. Under circumstances that allow the use of tissues and organs from persons who were murdered, it is **similarly allowable to use tissues and organs from fetuses who have been aborted . . .** , from **'excess' embryos** stored in *in vitro* fertilization clinics, **or from embryos that have been formed to produce tissues and organs**. The same can be said of knowledge derived from embryo and fetal research. There is **no bar in principle against using for a good end something that has been acquired by heinous means, as long as** one has **not been involved in** (1) **employing these evil means**, (2) **encouraging their use**, (3) **avoiding their condemnation**, or (4) **giving scandal through their use**. One can drink water from a well that was dug by unjustly forced labor.

That analysis poses three problems.

First, the analogies that he constructs in the first two sentences above at once unequal and morally irrelevant. Engelhardt equates the accidental deaths of a breathing person and a preborn child (i.e., a miscarriage) as sufficient cause for the morally licit use of tissues and organs, because there is no planned, willful, sinister act in either case. He deems as appropriate and moral the widespread practice today of transplanting (or, to use the common crass term, "harvesting") human organs pursuant to such unintended or non-culpable deaths.

However, a "miscarriage," though tragic to the mother and father of the lost baby, may pose a *sui generis* moral problem. *The Rudder*, the classic book of Orthodox canons (or rules for proper Orthodox behavior), includes a troubling canon pertaining to this subject by St. John the Faster, Patriarch of Constantinople (+ AD 595). His Canon 22 states, "A woman who involuntarily has expelled a baby through miscarriage receives her penance for a year."[25] To modern ears that may sound harsh and insensitive, and probably few Orthodox priests today would counsel a mother who lost her baby to refrain from the Holy Mysteries for a year. But St. John the Faster's insight about the sanctity of the miscarried child, I would suggest, ought to remind us that even such an involuntary death constitutes a loss of life of a unique, unrepeatable human person forever on this earth and give us pause, fourteen centuries later, before we hasten to "harvest" that innocent dead child's organs even for the benefit of other human beings. Orthodox Christianity has always insisted on proper reverential burial of the dead as intact as possible in anticipation of "the resurrection of the dead and the life of the age to come," as we profess whenever we recite the Niceno-Constantinopolitan Creed.

I would add, however, that two crucial caveats would preclude such a "harvesting" of organs in those circumstances even for those who do not concur with the view I expressed above: (1) prior documentary evidence that the deceased breathing person did not consent to any organ donation,

---

25. *The Rudder* (Pedalion), trans. D. Cummings (Chicago: The Orthodox Christian Educational Society, 1957), 99. (I thank my fellow priest and co-editor, Fr. Peter Heers, for reminding me about this canon.)

or (2) a decision by the surviving parent(s) of the deceased preborn baby to withhold parental consent to the practice.

Moreover, Engelhardt's subsequent comparison of the two types of accidental death to the murder of a breathing person and the murder (abortion) of a preborn child fails completely. Both murders are, unlike cases of accidental death, intrinsically unjust, evil acts perpetrated by agents freely and with full knowledge of what they are doing. Contrary to Engelhardt's analysis, I would oppose on moral grounds the "harvesting" of organs from either murdered victim. To be sure, in the case of the murdered born person who has enjoyed a measure of conscious human life, other Orthodox moral theologians, like Engelhardt, and many Orthodox faithful might be willing to condone an organ transplant if (1) the victim had not been murdered—whether in the first or second degree—precisely for the purpose of procuring one or more organs and (2) the next-of-kin authorized the procedure. However, a planned abortion always entails the methodical, medical destruction of a perfectly innocent, sinless human person in his or her mother's womb. Given the time sensitive exigencies of the harvesting of preborn baby organs, which must occur quickly before such organs atrophy, any abortion under those circumstances must necessarily have as one of its *conscious and willed* ends the *immediate* surgical removal of organs such as a kidney or a retina from the preborn baby. That is a calculated cold-blooded act of murder the enormity of which may have no equal in civilized societies.

Second, Engelhardt fortunately and properly puts "excess" in quotation marks when he refers to "'excess' embryos" stored in in vitro fertilization clinics, because human embryos are never "excess" or "unnecessary." But the phrases "fetuses who have been aborted" and "embryos that have been formed to produce tissues and organs" seem needlessly clinical and too detached. To be sure, Engelhardt is hardly alone even among Orthodox Christians in his choice of the word "fetus," and there are technical differences among the clinical terms zygote, embryo, and fetus pertaining to time of gestation in the mother's body. However, universal Orthodox moral tradition allows for no such distinctions in terms of abortion: the destruction of human life in the mother's body at any stage is equivalent to murdering an innocent human being. In this chapter and in my other publications, I have employed a more empathetic and theologically accurate term—namely, aborted preborn baby. In bioethics, as in much of contemporary scholarship and social life, he or she who controls the language has a better chance of prevailing in contentious ethical and political debates, as well as God willing, public policy. Orthodox moral theologians and bioethicists, above all others, ought to stand our ground in the "name game" and not yield an inch.

Third, and truly egregious, Engelhardt proposes a false teleology—indeed, a strictly secular, un-Orthodox utilitarian argument focused exclusively on the supposedly good intent of those who may wish "to use tissues and organs" from aborted preborn babies as a means to save human lives from deadly diseases with, however, total disregard for the evil intent that led to the willful, intrinsically evil action of abortion in the first place—that is, the needless, violent destruction of human persons that is the means or object of such abortions.

Engelhardt's confident proclamation that "there is no bar in principle against using for a good end something that has been acquired by heinous means" is, *prima facie*, a classic consequentialist mantra. His four enumerated conditions for licit use of aborted preborn baby cell lines toward the end of the excerpt above offer little nuance or value. The first seems to absolve anyone except the abortionists themselves and their collaborators who procured the desired cell lines; Engelhardt does not deem morally culpable those who utilize and benefit by the product of an abortion, even when they know the genesis of their bounty. The second condition is a non-sequitur. Anyone who freely benefits from such abortions provides a tacit *post-factum* encouragement of the original act and implicit permission for similar acts in the present and future. How can one in good conscience lay claim to the favorable consequences of a previous abortion, while precluding that same outcome for others in similar predicaments in the present? The third condition is effectively irrelevant. Even if a potential beneficiary condemns the evil of the original abortion(s), such a rejection of the original evil act does not absolve anyone from profiting from that act. Talk is cheap, as the saying goes. Finally, the question of "scandal" is self-evident. How anyone who utilizes aborted preborn baby cells or cell-lines even for a good end can avoid "giving scandal through their use" is beyond my comprehension, The "scandal" is inherent in the intrinsically evil act, and the hands of anyone who exploits that act are also dirty.

In fairness, I would also note that the very next sentence after the section of p. 261 quoted above might appear *prima facie* to qualify Engelhardt's otherwise utilitarian argument:

> However, one must be very careful neither to endorse nor to encourage any illicit circumstances or means. . . . Great spiritual discernment will be needed, and any use of such materials must at the very least

be approached penitentially as a concession to human weakness. After all, the postponement of death and the pursuit of health should never become all-consuming obsessions.

He sounds a proper cautionary note against obsessing about death and health, which underlies the intensity of public support for taking the COVID-19 vaccines in the first place. That intensity has now led to draconian decisions by various institutions—particularly colleges and universities, airlines, businesses, workplaces, and the U.S. armed forces— to mandate that anyone availing himself of those services or occupations take one of the current COVID-19 vaccines and provide tangible proof or suffer exclusion from that institution! The "choice" presented is a false one: conform, suffer exile, or become a social pariah. But it is still a daunting prospect for college students, frequent travelers, and others to refrain from the vaccines even on valid moral or religious grounds. Engelhardt's empathetic note ought to remind us that evil actions by anyone are subject to our personal moral assessment, but *we* are not, as Orthodox Christians, entitled to judge the *souls* of anyone we may deem morally errant.

Engelhardt's reference to "illicit circumstances or means" is precisely what is at stake in the moral analysis of this vaccine question. What I term illicit, Engelhardt pronounces licit. Moreover, he effectively, albeit unintentionally, concedes the moral argument altogether when he invokes "human weakness." Whether a moral actor is personally penitential for or indifferent to the act itself does not mitigate the objective enormity of the exploitation of aborted preborn baby cell lines in the development and testing of the COVID-19 vaccines. To appeal to "human weakness" in this case is, in effect, to blur the necessary distinctions and to concede the *moral* argument. The question of penitence is appropriate in Holy Confession, not on the operating table in a hospital or at the pharmacy, clinic, or abortion mill where the question is one of right or wrong.

Finally, it is fitting to consider a prophetic comment on p. 136 in Tristram Engelhardt's final book published a year before his death in 2018, titled *After God: Morality & Bioethics in a Secular Age*:

> [T]he central importance within the dominant secular culture of respect of persons is taken to require that one respect persons in their life- and death-style choices, however perverse and misguided these choices may be. That is, it is judged to be immoral to judge peaceable life- and death-style choices to be immoral, because one is required to respect persons in the choices that they are free to make within secular politics.[26]

> I offer the present chapter in that same spirit of judging moral choices and arguments without fear or timidity, but not the actors or proponents themselves.

C. OTSA's Group Statement

The Orthodox Theological Society in America (OTSA) released on March 8, 2021, a widely publicized public statement with this unwieldy title—"Covid-19 vaccines: How they are made and how they work to prime the immune system to fight SARS-CoV2."[27] OTSA is a voluntary guild

---

26. H. Tristram Engelhardt, *After God: Morality & Bioethics in a Secular Age* (Yonkers, NY: St. Vladimir's Seminary Press, 2017), 136.

27. https://www.otsamerica.net/wp-content/uploads/2021/03/Covid19-Vac-cineTech.pdf (Accessed on December 16, 2021).

of Orthodox scholars who hold "at least a Master's degree in theology (or its equivalent) or a master's degree in Arts, as well as significant additional graduate studies in theology or related disciplines."[28]

The OTSA statement prepared by Hermina Nedelescu, Ph.D., Catherine Creticos, M.D., and Gayle E. Woloschak, Ph.D., D.Min., provides a seeming patina of legitimacy to an ethical argument that ought to be abhorrent to any informed, devout Orthodox Christian. The statement declares boldly, "Most Church leaders have agreed that the many lives saved by vaccination are an important factor in permitting the use of these vaccines." It provides, however, links only to two Roman Catholic documents and a Zoom video of the "Halki IV" summit sponsored by the Patriarchate of Constantinople in January 2021. For the latter, the OTSA document states timidly, "Metropolitan Nathanael touches upon this question." However, the Greek Orthodox bishop of Chicago barely "touches" on the question in that video and appears hesitant and uncertain of his own position.

Here are the three most pertinent sections of that document with my interlinear comments and rebuttals in view of the length of those sections (boldface added for emphasis; my comments in italics within brackets).

"3. Have the mRNA vaccines relied on fetal cells at any point? Answer: The Pfizer and mRNA vaccines (as well as the not yet approved Novavax and Inovio vaccines) were not made from fetal cells that came from aborted fetuses. The

---

28. *Full disclosure:* I resigned as a member of OTSA after a group "vote" in 1998 in favor of the ecumenical Aleppo Statement calling for a "common Easter" among all Christians by AD 2001 that ignored the historic post-Passover timing of Pascha in Orthodox tradition.

vaccines were **tested in culture against fetal cells to help ensure that they would not harm a fetus**

[NOTE: *A disingenuous claim at best, since the harm to the original "fetus"—whether "wanted" or "unwanted", whether healthy or not—already occurred decades ago when her retinal cells were harvested for development of such vaccines; moreover, the integral testing phase of those vaccines relied on cell lines derived from those original cells.*]

as well as **to ensure that the technology works in a human cell**.

[NOTE: *"Works" well, that is, to reduce the cost of minimizing potential side-effects and to expedite the quick roll-out of these vaccines to a competitive market; hence the false "necessity" to utilize human cell lines derived from an aborted preborn baby.*]

These tests were done with cells derived from the **1960's and 1970's**

[NOTE: *Inaccurate dates: for HEK-293, a **kidney** cell line that was isolated from an aborted preborn baby in 1973 through "a routine induced abortion" of a "completely normal" baby, and for PER.C6, a **retinal** cell line —that is, from the **eye** of the preborn child—that was isolated from a "healthy fetus" at Leiden University in the Netherlands in 1985.*[29]]

from so-called **therapeutic** abortions.

[NOTE: *A weasel use of "therapeutic," which presumes some kind of medical situation: the specific abortions were planned and, therefore,*

---

29. Alvin Wong, MD, "The Ethics of HEK 293," *The National Catholic Bioethics Quarterly* 6:3 (Autumn 2006), 473-495: https://www.pdcnet.org/C1257D43006C9AB1/file/5 265B61D5497F52585257D94004802BB/$FILE/ncbq_2006_0006_0003_0077_0099. pdf, 473, 474, 475 (Accessed on December 16, 2021).

elective, and the aborted preborn babies were old enough in the womb to enable "harvesting" of organs such as their liver or eyes.[30]]

No new fetuses have been sacrificed since that time for any vaccine tests.

[NOTE: *A valid point but irrelevant to the sacrifice of the two aborted preborn babies who provided the original KEK-293 and PER. C6 cell lines.*].

In **contrast to** the mRNA vaccines, many of the other Covid-19 vaccines (e.g., AstraZeneca and Johnson & Johnson) are grown using the same fetal cell line. To 'grow' the vaccine in fetal cells is a term that scientists use because all viruses are dependent on cells for "growth," which for a virus means to replicate, and thus, the production of viral vaccines will require cells for production.

[NOTE: *Whether a vaccine was grown in, derived from, or tested with a fetal kidney or retinal cell is a distinction without a moral difference: the process is still connected to a heinous act of abortion.*]

Most vaccines do not 'grow' well in adult cells, and therefore **require the use of fetal cells**.

[NOTE: *Expedience is not a moral justification; moreover, other prospective COVID-19 vaccines still in development (see section III of this chapter below) do not utilize human cell-lines*]

Importantly, mRNA vaccines are synthesized without cells. Vaccine synthesis and vaccine production are two separate steps in the vaccine making pipeline. Some vaccines (e.g., Rubella, chickenpox) used in the United States also

---

30. https://www.lifesitenews.com/blogs/the-unborn-babies-used-for-vaccine-development-were-alive-at-tissue-extraction (Accessed on December 16, 2021).

come from viruses grown in aborted fetal cells (again, from those cells from the 1960's and 1970's). The United States government has banned the generation of any new cells or the sacrifice of any embryos for the purpose of investigation. **Nevertheless, it is recognized that some vaccines would not be possible without growth of the viral vaccines in these fetal cells**.

[NOTE: *Hence the moral argument against those vaccines.*]

"4. Are the vaccines unethical because of their use of aborted fetal cells? Answer: Several significant factors lead to the conclusion that the vaccines present the best ethical option to promote health and life, despite their connection with the use of aborted fetal cells. These factors are: (1) The fetal cells in use today are derived from two or three therapeutic abortions performed several decades ago. **The abortions were NOT for the purpose of the development of vaccines,**

[NOTE: *Perhaps not specifically at the times of the hideous "harvesting" of the desired cells, but the original abortions were, obviously, not natural miscarriages. Whatever intentions the scientists had when they sought the organs deemed necessary for their biomedical experiments, these do not mitigate, much less justify, the original abortion abomination. Nor are anyone's hands who was connected in any way to those abortions—from the willing mother to the attending medical personnel and the scientists— morally clean.*]

and all parties (including the US government) have agreed that **no new fetuses** will be aborted or used for this purpose...

[NOTE: *Thank God for that, but the two "original sins" that occurred in the 1970s and 1980s remain in effect and continue to stain the souls of those who choose to benefit from them.*]

(2) Many vaccines (other than COVID) that we use in the US and world-wide are made from these cells, and other substitute cell lines have not proven to be effective for growing the vaccines; this has been **the only alternative**.

[NOTE: *False! Only some, if any, vaccines are derived from these cells. Again, see section III below for new or forthcoming viable alternatives.*]

(3) Most Church leaders have agreed that the many lives saved by vaccination are an important factor in permitting the use of these vaccines. While it is a sad reality that the origin of these cell lines is from these **very few therapeutic abortions**,

[NOTE: *No Orthodox theologian should employ the artificial medical distinction between "elective" abortion—that is, for any reason—and "therapeutic" abortion—that is, for a woman with a special health condition. Orthodox moral tradition since the earliest Church Fathers in the second century has universally opposed abortions for any reason.*]

the **cell lines are already in existence**,

[NOTE: *A non-sequitur that glosses over the original intrinsic evil entailed in procuring those cell lines.*]

no new fetuses will be used, and as such it is **far preferable**

[NOTE: *A meaningless comparative: it is never licit and not even "necessary" in view of the imminent availability of alternative vaccines without abortion pedigrees. See section III below. Moreover, when the current cell lines lose their efficacy, would OTSA and others who support the current COVID-19 vaccines resort to the same immoral argument by "necessity" and validate new cell lines derived from fresh abortions?*]

to cure diseases as a result of the use of these cell lines than to totally forbid the use of these cell lines. **The vaccines in no way legitimize or promote abortion**;

[NOTE: *A disingenuous claim at best: exploiting the consequences of an abortion, particularly cells extracted from the preborn baby, entails a material sharing of the guilt for the original abomination and provides tacit approval for similar exploitations in the present or future, claims to the contrary notwithstanding.*]

rather they combat disease and death, support health, and enable life—not death—to prevail, all of which are of **the highest ethical value**.

[NOTE: *That argument focuses narrowly on the ostensibly moral ends alone and fails to take seriously the evil means presumed necessary to those ends—namely, the original abortions, whose preborn baby "donors" were unable to consent to the organ "harvesting" in the first place, and who were victims of objectively, intrinsically evil acts akin to similar abominations on a mass scale such as the slaughter of innocent beings in genocides including the Holocaust. Does the "highest" ethical choice favor one's own life at the expense of another's?*]

More information regarding the morality of using these cell lines can be found at the following links:
(1) Ecumenical Patriarchate—"Halki Summit IV—Covid-19 and Climate change: Living with and Learning from a Pandemic." **Metropolitan Nathanael** touches upon this question.

[NOTE: *Of the Greek Orthodox Archdiocese, not the Romanian Episcopate of the Orthodox Church in America.*]

https://www.facebook.com/ ecumenicalpatriarchate/videos/900946820672806/

(2) The Vatican – Congregation for the Doctrine of the Faith https://www.vatican.va/roman_curia/ congregations/cfaith/documents/rc_con_cfaith_ doc_20201221_not a-vaccini-anticovid_en.html

(3) United States Conference of Catholic Bishops https://www.usccb.org/moral-considerations-covid-vaccines

[NOTE: *That is a very selective use of sources in agreement with OTSA's statement.*]

5. Some new COVID vaccines (such as Johnson and Johnson) are grown in fetal cells. Are these vaccines, in particular, unethical, and should we avoid them? Answer: No. Although the use of "more" fetal cells in one type of vaccine than another (for example, by growing the vaccine in the cells as opposed to simply testing them using the cell line) appears **to suggest that more fetal deaths occurred or that more fetuses were involved**, this is NOT accurate.

[NOTE: *A deflection tactic: no one I know is making that claim. The use of aborted preborn baby cells, an easier task compared to utilizing cell lines, simply positions Johnson and Johnson more closely to the original abortion abomination.*]

All the cells used are clones from the same original fetal cell lines, and whether a few cells or many are used, there are NO new fetuses involved. The ethics of taking one vaccine is essentially no different from that of another.

[*NOTE: False! Even the two original cell lines required numerous experiments involving many more aborted babies to prove useful for the COVID-19 vaccines. OTSA fails to mention COVID-19 vaccines in development—such as CVnCoV (CureVac's mRNA-based vaccine candidate in Germany). See section III below.]*

II. Orthodox Hierarchs and Synods in Opposition

On the other side of the question—and yes, two distinct, mutually exclusive moral worldviews in the worldwide Orthodox Church are at stake—are at least six unequivocal documents produced by Orthodox hierarchs and synods around the globe (boldface added for emphasis).

First, chapter 12, section 7, of the Bases of the Social Concept of the Russian Orthodox Church (AD 2000), an extraordinary and reliable, for the most part, compendium of moral analyses of a multitude of issues approved by the Holy Synod of the Patriarchate of Moscow, includes this unequivocal, morally consistent position, which stands in stark contrasts to the frantic expediency that drives the positions of the three Russian Orthodox hierarchs discussed above (boldface in original text):

> **The Church believes it to be definitely inadmissible to use the methods of so-called foetal therapy** in which the human foetus on various stages of its development is aborted and used in attempts to treat various diseases and to 'rejuvenate' an organism. Denouncing abortion as a cardinal sin, the Church cannot find any justification for it either even if someone may possibly benefit from the destruction of a conceived human life. Contributing inevitably to ever wider spread and commercialization of abortion, this practice (even if its still hypothetical effectiveness could

be proved scientifically) presents an example of glaring immorality and is criminal.[31]

Second, a press release on "The Cloning of Embryonic Cells" by the Holy Synod of the Church of Greece on August 17, 2000, in the aftermath of the successful experimental cloning of a sheep in the United Kingdom named "Dolly," included this ringing denunciation of human cloning through the use "human embryonic cells" derived from abortions (boldface added for emphasis):

> The recent decision of the British Government to permit experimentation on human embryonic cells derived from cloning of the Dolly type, triggered an intense political and medical dispute, which also reopens the need to emphasize that **the ethical criterion is incomparably higher than any scientific achievement**...
>
> Whereupon:
>
> a) Our Church expresses her **explicit opposition to conducting experiments on human embryonic cells. What is named thus implies the destruction not of embryonic cells but human embryos.**
>
> b) The position that the human person begins to develop from the 14th day after conception offers an alibi to British scientists, but this, having a scholastic derivation and not a scientific basis, consists of subjective belief and arbitrary opinion. The Church

---

31. http://orthodoxeurope.org/page/3/14.aspx (Accessed on December 16, 2021).

and Christian conscience accept the human being as person [πρόσωπο] with an eternal and timeless perspective from the moment of conception.

c) Differentiations [distinctions/discriminations] between people are continuously increasing. **Everything indicates that the course of our societies is clearly all the more "eugenics" and racist. An attempt, however, to improve life cannot pass through the destruction of millions of human beings of embryonic [fetal] age**[32]

It is at once disappointing and tragic that the recent statements by the same Holy Synod of Greece explicitly endorsing the current COVID-19 vaccines discussed earlier in this chapter contradict and undermine the wisdom of those bishops in AD 2000.

Third, a section on "The Transplant of Organs" on the Official Site of the Romanian Patriarchate lists these mandatory "principles," among others, for proper, moral utilization of human organs and tissues, which collectively point to a rejection of the "harvesting" of aborted preborn baby organs to extract cells for any purpose without the consent of the preborn child-victim—an obvious impossibility—even to save the life of someone, which is, of course, the stated purpose of those who support the current COVID-19 vaccines:

---

32. https://www.bioethics.org.gr/03_c.html#6 (Accessed on July 16, 2021). Translation of the Greek original by Protopresbyter George A. Alexson (Ashburn, Virginia).

- Because the extraction of organs implies the consent of the donor, extraction of tissues from an embryo is unconceivable given the fact that although alive, this one cannot give its consent.
- It is not admitted to cause mutilation or death through the extraction of organs, even to save the life of another person.
- The Church cannot agree with the transplant of the embryoid tissues which involves the risk to affect the good health of the fetus and neither with using the transplant of the organs of the acephalous or hydrocephalous newborn (sic) babies.[33]

Fourth, though not as pointed in their opposition to the COVID-19 on the substance of the issue as the autocephalous Orthodox Church of Romania, the Holy Synod of the semi-autonomous Moldovan Orthodox Church of the Moscow Patriarchate (in the primarily Romanian-speaking southwest corner of the Russian Federation), noting that "an increasing number of presidents, politicians, deputies, businessmen and medical experts openly declare testing of certain vaccines against COVID-19, which should be mandatory" (sic), appealed publicly to the governing authorities in Moldova on May 19, 2020: "[V]accination of the population, as well as any medical intervention, should be carried out on a voluntary basis, only with the consent and full information of the patient."[34]

---

33. http://patriarhia.ro/transplant-of-organs-6021-en.html (Accessed on December 16, 2021). Unfortunately, that statement did not go far enough. See the discussion above re the dubious practice of "harvesting" human organs under any circumstances, as well as footnote 26.

34. "Vaccines Must Be Optional, Moldovan Church Tells State Authorities":

Fifth, in a joint public letter on August 21, 2020, to Scott Morrison, Prime Minister of Australia, the Anglican Archbishop Glen Davies of Sydney, Roman Catholic Archbishop Anthony Fisher of Sydney, and Archbishop Makarios (Griniezakis), Primate of the Greek Orthodox Archdiocese of Australia, tried to distance themselves, on moral grounds, from any vaccines derived from "fetal cell lines"—that is, from aborted preborn babies. Here are the key points of their public defense of those people of faith who would reject certain COVID-19 vaccines on moral grounds even before the initial group of vaccines became available in 2021:

> Some will have no ethical problem with using tissue from electively aborted foetuses for medical purposes. Others may regard the use of a cell-line derived from an abortion performed back in the 1970s as now sufficiently removed from the abortion itself to be excusable. But others again will draw a straight line from the ending of a human life in abortion through the cultivation of the cell-line to the use for manufacturing this vaccine; even if the cells have been propagated for years in a laboratory far removed from the abortion, that line of connection remains. They will be concerned not to benefit in any way from the death of the little girl whose cells were taken and cultivated, nor to be trivializing that death, and not to be encouraging the foetal tissue industry.
>
> While we accept that the proposed vaccine may be sufficiently remote from the abortion that occasioned

the derivation of the cell-line, we flag to you that any COVID-19 vaccine cultured on a foetal cell-line will raise serious issues of conscience for a proportion of our population. Those troubled by this may either acquiesce to the social and political pressure to use the vaccine, or conscientiously object to the use by themselves and their dependents; if the latter, they will suffer various disadvantages (e.g., denial of access to childcare, aged care or employment) . . .

The three archbishops then, noting that "other vaccine trials . . . do not involve the use of morally compromised fetal cell lines," seek assurance from their Australian government that the latter will not compel those citizens who have "conscientious or moral" objections to take any vaccine connected to fetal cell lines and "will ensure that an ethically uncontroversial alternative vaccine be made available in Australia if it is achieved."[35]

Sixth, in his own prophetic "Archpastoral Reflection on Current Covid Crisis" updated on September 15, 2021, Bishop Silouan of the Serbian Orthodox Metropolitanate of Australia and New Zealand, cited the bold public moral witness by the three Australian cosignatories of the ecumenical letters quoted above and offers himself as an authoritative reference for those seeking religious exemptions from COVID-19 vaccines mandated by any earthly authorities:

Orthodox Christians . . . have a moral issue accepting vaccines that have been developed from cell lines that

---

35. Full text available at https://www.9news.com.au/national/coronavirus-vaccine-archbishops-raise-ethical-concerns-over-foetal-cell-lines/bd212356-abef-44b7-853a-130b2ac648b2 (Accessed on December 16, 2021).

were obtained from tissues harvested from aborted fetuses. The issue of ethical concerns for such vaccines was raised last year by some of the major Christian jurisdictions in Australia, such as the Roman Catholic, the Anglican and Greek Orthodox Archdioceses.

Therefore, the moral concerns of Christians should be taken into consideration, as they are not simply subjective views, but derive from the fundamental positions and core beliefs of the Church.

That is why our faithful may appeal to this, our Archpastoral letter, and other statements of the Orthodox Church as to why they are unable to receive these particular vaccines.[36]

Seventh, also in Australia (our Lord has raised up some wonderful prophets "down under" during this crisis!), Bishop George (Schaefer) of Canberra, Auxiliary Bishop of the Australian & New Zealand Diocese of the Russian Orthodox Church Outside Russia, issued an encyclical on August 5, 2021, which is the strongest unequivocal, courageous, unambiguous, and pastoral (in the best sense of that often misused term) condemnation of the current COVID-19 vaccines on moral grounds to date among the worldwide hierarchy of the Church. Here is the most significant section:

> There are some Orthodox hierarchs who condone taking the vaccines, even though they contain fetal cells, or are derived from fetal cells, thereby being a direct product of abortion. In good conscience, as an Orthodox Christian, I cannot agree with this view and

---

36. Full text available at https://soc.org.au/en/news/1519-archpastoral-reflection-on-current-covid-crisis (Accessed on December 16, 2021).

cannot condone it. However, considering that there are some Orthodox hierarchs who do allow these vaccines, and considering the great fear campaign that is being waged by the governments and the media, I can understand if people do decide to get vaccinated. People also need to know that many of those who are getting vaccinated are dying or experiencing severe side effects. We must be aware of what we are doing. Whatever our personal choice is in this matter, we must still live as Orthodox Christians, loving and encouraging one another, being an example of Christian love and piety both to those in our Church communities and to others. Let us re-focus our priorities and focus more on our own spiritual life, not just on preserving our physical life in this sinful world, so when the time comes that God summons us to the next life, we may be able to give a good account of our life here on earth, time in which we should be repenting and preparing ourselves spiritually for eternity.[37]

In a subsequent official letter on September 15, 2021, addressed to Gladys Berejeklian, Premier of the New South Wales Province, and The Hon. Daniel Andrews, Premier of the Victoria Province in Australia, Bishop George of Canberra also manned the prophet's mantle and took square aim at mandatory COVID-19 vaccine "passports," or printed proof of a person's vaccination against COVID-19, which

---

37. Full text available at https://www.rocor.org.au/news10/wp-content/uploads/2021/08/Epistle-English-5-August-2021.pdf (Accessed on December 16, 2021).

are already proving abhorrent to the civil liberties of many on either moral side of the COVID-19 vaccine controversy:

> Vaccine passports will create a two-tiered society and we strongly condemn this proposed measure. The Church CANNOT enforce such discriminatory measures in our parishes and refuse entry to anybody who seeks to attend without the proposed vaccine passport, or any other certificate, as this would lead to discriminatory outcomes and violate the Church's teachings and canons.
>
> In our multicultural and multi-faith society, these proposed measures, which are divisive, coercive, and discriminatory, echo the trials experienced by many before they fled persecution and now call Australia home.
>
> We implore and pray that you—our elected leaders— are made aware of the terrible consequences of such an unethical measure. History is the best teacher on where such courses of action have to in the past.[38]

Serbian Orthodox Bishop Silouan (cited above) also included in his public missive on September 15, 2021— the same day as Bishop George—this at once prophetic and pastoral pledge to his flock regarding the mandated COVID-19 "passports"

---

38. Full text available at https://www.rocor.org.au/news10/wp-content/uploads/2021/09/Open-letter-passport-Sept21.pdf and https://www.pokrov.com.au/news-and-events/australia-and-new-zealand-diocese-response-to-vaccine-passport (Accessed on December 16, 2021). Bishop Silouan of the Serbian Orthodox Church also condemned the "Vaccine Passport" in his Archpastoral Letter.

I would also like to mention as a great concern the alarming prospects of the introduction of Vaccine Passports. I believe that this will lead to a two-tiered society, it will divide people, families, and friends and will provide a basis for acts of discrimination and ostracization.

In relation to this, media reports have also mentioned that "Churches will be required to use Vaccination Certificate Systems for Vaccinated-ONLY Worship"?!?

This is totally foreign to the Spirit of the Church, to the ecclesiology, the Holy Gospel and Tradition of the Church. We could never accept or adopt such a practice! It would entail discrimination against those who are members of the same Body, The Body of Christ, His Holy Church. How can we go against the Gospel? Against Christ who exclaims: "Come to Me, all you who labour and are heavy laden, and I will give you rest" (Mathew 11:28).

We cannot accept the polarisation of the faithful, it goes against the very nature of the Church, and we will not be implementing this system in our churches.

The Church embraces all who seek Christ, those vaccinated and unvaccinated. It will seek to heal a wounded and heavy-laden society, not inflict new wounds and burdens.[39]

Eighth, one more Orthodox hierarch deserves special attention as the only one in North America, so far, who has stepped forward and proclaimed the full Orthodox moral tradition pertaining to the COVID-19 crisis. On October

---

39. Full text available at https://soc.org.au/en/news/1519-archpastoral-reflection-on-current-covid-crisis (Accessed on December 16, 2021).

29, 2021, Metropolitan Jonah (Paffhausen), former primate of the Orthodox Church in America, retired bishop in the Russian Orthodox Church Outside Russia, and rector of St. Herman of Alaska Russian Orthodox Church in Stafford, Virginia, since 2017, offered the following comprehensive statement on the key issues:

> The Covid vaccine is one among a whole set of issues, which have both religious and legal, as well as moral implications.
>
> The primary religious concern is the outright moral case against the use of fetal cells from aborted babies to develop the vaccines. This implies the validation of abortion, and the use of the fetuses killed during those procedures for medical and testing purposes. For an Orthodox or Catholic Christian, the implicit validation of abortion is utterly immoral. Thus, the use of vaccines developed with such cells is not only immoral, but a mortal sin.
>
> The Orthodox Church in America and Russian Orthodox Church, among others, have explicitly condemned use of fetal cells in medical testing. The products of those experiments are under the same ban.
>
> On the political or social level, to have a vaccine mandated by the government is a basic offense against personal sovereignty over one's own body. While many people may not care about the moral component, the vaccine as mandated by the U.S. administration forces the violation of the integrity of the body. This violation of personal freedom and sovereignty over oneself is itself a moral violation of one's personhood.

That the vaccine is not fully tested and approved, is not a traditional vaccine but experimental gene therapy, and has many serious side effects further places the vaccine in a dubious light. That this is government mandated, with very serious consequences for non-compliance, should compel society to make the vaccine a matter of individual free personal choice. Otherwise, the U.S. government is in violation of the Fourth Amendment to the U.S. Constitution, which guarantees that citizens of the United States be secure in their persons.

The mandates are problematic because, first, they deprive people of their right to work and, therefore, of their livelihoods and, second, they preclude their ability to participate in society and in the economy, to enter restaurants, stores and public places. The issue is not that they are any more a danger to public health than fully vaccinated individuals. Rather, the "unvaccinated" are being punished severely because they are politically non-compliant. Not only is this unconscionable as a form of totalitarian control; it has dire religious implications. That people would be forbidden to buy and sell without the mark of compliance to the government is apocalyptic. By imposing that mandate the U.S. administration identifies itself with the Beast of Revelation.[40]

---

40. Personal email to me, October 29, 2021.

III. Morally Licit Vaccines on the Horizon?

Thanks to the providence of God the Holy Trinity, conscientious Orthodox Christians do not confront a zero-sum moral decision between any or all COVID-19 vaccines or no COVID-19 vaccines. Some Orthodox Christians, together with other Americans, may have serious doubts or objections to many or all COVID-19 vaccines for practical or medical reasons such as imminent death, debilitating or life-threatening side effects, unpublicized biological manipulation of recipients' bodies, or possible violations of privacy by tracking or controlling devices that may be inherent in the vaccines.[41] These concerns are beyond the scope of my argument in this chapter, which addresses the primary moral issues alone.

Several COVID-19 vaccines still in development have no connections to aborted preborn baby cells or cell lines. The website of the Charlotte Lozier Institute provides a link (updated as recently as June 2, 2021) to a widely-circulated chart of which vaccines do and which do not utilize such cells or cell lines and to what extent: https://lozierinstitute.org/update-covid-19-vaccine-candidates-and-abortion-derived-cell-lines/. The vaccines in development, marked exclusively with green squares, are potentially good moral alternatives to those unacceptable vaccines that OTSA and many Orthodox hierarchs have blessed. To be sure, the

---

41. See, for example, Jon Cohen, "Further evidence supports controversial claim that SARS-CoV-2 genes can integrate with human DNA," May, 6, 2021: https://www.sciencemag.org/news/2021/05/further-evidence-offered-claim-genes-pandemic-coronavirus-can-integrate-human-dna (Accessed on December 16, 2021).

virtue of prudence may preclude any vaccines produced in Communist China, above all the one in development at the infamous Wuhan Institute, the source of the COVID-19 virus in the first place.

Two vaccines still in the mid-phases of development utilize "Vero" cell lines derived from the kidney of an African green monkey dating back to 1962 instead of aborted preborn human baby cells: the vaccine from Osaka University— AnGes, Takara Bio—in Japan and the vaccine from the Israel Institute for Biological Research (IIBR).

Two other vaccines have completed all phases of development and testing and will be imminently available to selected nations. The BBV152 vaccine known as COVAXIN from the Bharat Biotech/Indian Council of Medical Research in India is most promising, because it meets all moral and religious objections.[42] According to the host website, the COVAXIN vaccine is an "indigenous, inactivated vaccine" that was "developed using **Whole-Virion Inactivated Vero Cell** derived platform technology. Inactivated vaccines do not replicate and are therefore unlikely to revert and cause pathological effects. They contain dead virus, incapable of infecting people but still able to instruct the immune system to mount a defensive reaction against an infection."[43]

Fellow Orthodox theologian and active U.S. Navy chaplain Fr. Andrew Kearns shared with me this excellent prospect in a personal email on August 20, 2021:

---

42. Charlotte Lozier Institute: https://lozierinstitute.org/update-covid-19-vaccine-candidates-and-abortion-derived-cell-lines/ (Accessed on December 16, 2021).

43. Bharat Biotech: https://www.bharatbiotech.com/covaxin.html (Accessed on December 16, 2021).

While Covaxin distribution in the US is currently hindered by legal matters concerning Ocugen, the company with the rights to distribute in North America, this vaccine has completed Phase 1-3 trials and has emergency authorization in 16 countries. It should also be receiving WHO emergency authorization soon and is still in the process of being reviewed for FDA approval.

That vaccine may be available nearby in Mexico soon.

Another alternative vaccine might have been CVnCoV, the product of a collaboration between CureVac and Bayer AG in Germany and the GlaxoSmithKline (GSK) pharma group in the United Kingdom. (That is the same Bayer pharmaceutical company that has supplied aspirins to American families for decades.) The CureVac COVID-19 vaccine had completed all phases of development and testing. Its manufacture and initial distribution in the 27 member nations of the European Union by CureVac (Germany) and Novartis (Austria) was slated for "late summer 2021."[44] However, an official press release on October 12, 2021, datelined Tubingen, Germany, and Boston, USA, announced that the CVnCoV vaccine would be "withdrawn from regulatory review" and retooled as a "second-generation" COVID-19 vaccine, estimating "that the earliest potential approval of CVnCoV would come in the second quarter of

---

44. For details see https://www.biopharma-reporter.com/Article/2021/03/22/CureVac-on-track-to-apply-for-COVID-19-vaccine-market-authorization-in-Q2-2021 and https://www.biopharma-reporter.com/Article/2021/02/03/GSK-and-CureVac-in-tie-up-to-address-multiple-emerging-variants-with-one-COVID-19-vaccine (Accessed on December 16, 2021).

2022."[45] Why the delay? An earlier press release on June 30, 2021, revealed the disappointing data from the Phase 2b/3 Trial of the vaccine, specifically a "Vaccine efficacy of 48% against COVID-19 of any severity across all age groups and 15 variants."[46] Those test results remind us that the sound science of vaccines may entail a long period of development, production, and testing and ought never to be rushed unlike the full complement of current COVID-19 vaccines.

The CVnCoV may still be worth considering in the long term. It is a "non-replicating mRNA" vaccine by which "cell machinery is used to make a specific viral antigen and once this is accomplished, the mRNA is cleared," unlike other prospective COVID-19 vaccines that are "self-replicating (or self-amplifying) RNA vaccines," which provide "for abundant production of viral antigen" that remain in the body.[47]

---

45. https://www.curevac.com/en/2021/10/12/curevac-to-shift-focus-of-covid-19-vaccine-development-to-second-generation-mrna-technology/ (Accessed on December 16, 2021).

46. https://www.curevac.com/en/2021/06/30/curevac-final-data-from-phase-2b-3-trial-of-first-generation-covid-19-vaccine-candidate-cvncov-demonstrates-protection-in-age-group-of-18-to-60/ (Accessed on December 16, 2021).

47. For an understandable scientific explanation, see https://www.publichealthontario.ca/-/media/documents/ncov/vaccines/2020/12/covid-19-mrna-vaccines.pdf?la=en (Accessed on December 16, 2021). However, an alarming claim from the Doctors for Covid Ethics group chaired by Sucharit Bhakdi, MD, Professor Emeritus of Medical Microbiology and Immunology, Johannes Gutenberg University of Mainz (Germany), that raises concerns about potentially deadly "antibody-dependent enhancement" (ADE) in the Moderna mRNA-1273 vaccine specifically is worthy of serious consideration: "Letter to Physicians: Four New Scientific Discoveries Regarding the Safety and Efficacy of COVID-19 Vaccines": https://jamesfetzer.org/2021/07/letter-to-physicians-four-new-scientific-discoveries-regarding-the-safety-and-efficacy-of-covid-19-vaccines/ (Accessed on December 16, 2021).

And yet there is another obstacle for Orthodox and other Americans. The quantity of available CureVac vaccines would be limited to one hundred million doses per annum with only fifty million available through its initial months of distribution.[48] CureVac was and still would be intended for areas around the globe without alternative COVID-19 vaccines. That would exclude the United States and Canada for the immediate future. If the second-generation CureVac vaccine becomes available, direct appeals to the CureVac authorities by Americans and Canadians with profound religious objections to the current batch of vaccines but no objection to mRNA vaccines in principle might persuade the German company to provide directly at cost their morally acceptable vaccine as an exception to their current policy.

In short, "hope is on the way" for those conscientious objectors to the morally unacceptable vaccines currently available who have no qualms about travelling to Mexico for the COVAXIN vaccine from India or waiting for the mRNA CureVac vaccine from Germany—*if* those faithful Orthodox can stay the course and resist the temptation to settle now for instant medical mammon.

IV. The Moral Argument Against Most COVID-19 Vaccines

To summarize my moral case against *all* the COVID-19 vaccines currently available and *most* still in production,

---

48. https://www.curevac.com/en/2021/03/30/celonic-and-curevac-an-nounce-agreement-to-manufacture-over-100-million-doses-of-curevacs-covid-19-vaccine-candidate-cvncov/ (Accessed on December 16, 2021).

I offer the following reflections as one Orthodox moral theologian—no more, no less.

We must reject, on moral grounds, all COVID-19 vaccines that have *any* connection to aborted preborn baby cells or cell lines (especially from those babies in the second trimester of gestation who were "kept alive" long enough during the abortion procedure for scientists to extract the kidneys or retinas from which they derived the desired "material.") Time and distance are irrelevant to profiteering from such abominations for any reason, including the possible saving of human lives in the present or future. According to traditional Orthodox moral theology (as opposed to revisionist deviations so widespread today) beginning with several biblical proscriptions—namely, 3 John 11 and Romans 12:17, 12:21, and 3:8—certain actions ("means" to "ends") are objectively or intrinsically evil under *any* "circumstances"—most notably, abortion, rape, child abuse, incest, adultery, fornication, homosexual activity, physical torture of prisoners, and deliberate targeting of non-combatants in war.

Otherwise, we fall into a utilitarian or, worse, consequentialist temptation that justifies anything, however repellent, abominable, and otherwise deemed an evil, for the "greater good" that one may have as his or her intention. The New Testament, the *consensus patrum*, and our own properly Orthodox-informed consciences all testify to the uncontestable moral maxim that we may not do evil to achieve good. There is no "lesser evil" that is tolerable to achieve a "greater good." If the means or action toward even a good end is intrinsically evil, the entire decision is inescapably immoral, against conscience, and forbidden. A "lesser evil" decision process cloaked in a "greater good" teleology is either dangerous sophistry or *prelest*.

In the grand scheme of things, this pandemic is only one of numerous, more deadly pandemics in history. Despite the death tolls—each one a sorrowful loss for loved ones left behind—is our own bodily health, including immunity via vaccination, worth compromising an informed moral conscience by benefiting in any way from the abomination of abortion?

Alas, we confront in the third decade of the 21st century an omnipresent use of aborted preborn baby cells or cell lines in a wide variety of medical vaccines as well as comparatively trivial consumer items such as cosmetics and certain foods.

On October 30, 2009, Neocutis, a cosmetics company based in San Francisco, issued a statement defending its use of skin tissue from an aborted 14-week-old male baby to produce anti-aging creams: "Our view—which is shared by most medical professionals and patients—is that the limited, prudent and responsible use of donated fetal skin tissue can continue to ease suffering, speed healing, save lives and improve the well-being of many patients around the globe."[49]

While dismissing the occasional charge that some vaccines and other products contain actual cells from recent abortions, the McGill University Office for Science and Society in Canada—no friend of the pro-life movement— had to concede the following: "Senomyx, an American biotechnology company develops flavour enhancers for use in food products. To evaluate these enhancers, they used

---

49. Quoted in "Aborted Fetus Cells Used in Beauty Creams," The Washington Times, November 3, 2009: https://www.washingtontimes.com/news/2009/nov/3/aborted-fetus-cells-used-in-anti-aging-products/ (Accessed on December 16, 2021).

taste receptors expressed in the HEK 293 cell line, which was generated from the kidney cells of a fetus aborted in 1973."[50]

On September 13, 2021, the Conway Regional Hospital in Little Rock, Arkansas, erected a new hurdle for those who oppose the current COVID-19 vaccines for moral or religious reasons. CEO and President of Conway Regional Hospital, Matt Troup, announced a unique requirement that its employees who wish to request a religious exemption from the current COVID-19 vaccines must also *certify in writing* that those employees will not take any of thirty "everyday medicines" that also utilized aborted preborn baby cell lines at one stage or another of their development. Included among those medicines are popular products such as acetaminophen, albuterol, aspirin, ibuprofen, Tylenol, Pepto Bismol, Tums, Lipitor, Senokot, Motrin, Maalox, Ex-Lax, Benadryl, Sudafed, Preparation H, Claritin, Prilosec, and Zoloft.[51]

The first major problem with that maneuver is that Matt Troup plays fast and loose with the facts. For example, aspirin was created in 1897, Tylenol in 1886 (and first tested on human beings in 1893), Pepto-Bismol in 1901, Ex-Lax in

---

50. Ada McVein, "Is It True That Perfumes Contain Aborted Fetal Tissue?" March 22, 2019: https://www.mcgill.ca/oss/article/test-you-asked/it-true-per-fumes-contain-aborted-fetal-tissue (Accessed on December 16, 2021).

51. See the KARK TV, Little Rock, Arkansas website for the news story and a screen shot of Matt Troup's official letter and a list of all thirty medicines: https://www.kark.com/news/health/coronavirus/arkansas-hospital-lets-staff-seek-vaccine-exemption-as-long-as-they-dont-use-other-meds-tested-on-fetal-cell-lines/ (Accessed on December 16, 2021).

1906, and Tums in 1928, to name only five of the medicines in Troup's widely circulated list.[52]

In an article published in The National Catholic Bioethics Quarterly in 2006 that has gained a wide audience since the COVID-19 crisis in 2020, Alvin Wong, MD, provided a pertinent timeline:

> The use of aborted fetuses in the development of cell lines had begun as early as the sixties, looking at the well-known WI-38 and MRC-5 lines. The WI-38 cell line was developed in July 1962 from lung tissue taken from a therapeutically aborted fetus of about three months' gestational age, while the MRC-5 cell line was developed in September 1966 from lung tissue taken from a fourteen-week-old fetus aborted for psychiatric reasons from a twenty-seven-year-old physically healthy woman.[53]

That leaves us with the year 1962 as the *terminus a quo* for the exploitation of aborted preborn babies for cells converted into cell lines. Let's concede, to expedite the argument, Hans Clevers' claim of an earlier date for medical and pharmaceutical exploitation of aborted baby cells and cell lines than the HEK cell line: "Fetal tissue has been used for research in the U.S. since the 1930s, with bipartisan support from the Congress and funding from the National

---

52. Suzan Sammons, "Stop Pretending the COVID Jab is Morally Equivalent to Other Meds," *Crisis Magazine*, September 7, 2021: https://www.crisismagazine.com/2021/stop-pretending-the-covid-jab-is-morally-equivalent-to-other-meds (Accessed on December 16, 2021).

53. Alvin Wong, MD, "The Ethics of HEK 293," *The National Catholic Bioethics Quarterly* 6:3 (Autumn 2006), 475-476: https://www.pdcnet.org/C1257D43006C9AB1/file/5265B61D5497F52585257D94004802BB/$FILE/ncbq_2006_0006_0003_0077_0099.pdf, (Accessed on December 16, 2021).

Institutes of Health."[54] The 1930 date cited by Clevers still precludes the five medicines listed by Troup above from any possible use of aborted preborn baby cells or cell lines for their development, production, or testing simply because the technology was not yet invented![55]

A more serious challenge to Troup's pontifical decision for his hospital in Arkansas takes square aim at his faulty reasoning. The historical and scientific facts aside, this new standard of moral "consistency" may seem at once daunting and beguiling. But it entails a logical fallacy. A person need not be perfectly consistent and decline to use any of those meds—if, in fact, each of them did utilize aborted preborn baby cell lines, which now is dubious—just as a person may oppose a particular war on moral grounds as unjust without

---

54. Hans Clevers, "Fetal tissue research is essential for scientific discovery and improving human health," Oct. 5, 2017: https://www.statnews.com/2017/10/05/fetal-tissue-research-congress-nih/ (Accessed on December 16, 2021).

55. For a longer list of 42 prescription and over-the-counter medications supposedly connected to aborted preborn baby cells or cell lines, see Fr. Matthew Schneider, "If Any Drug Tested on HEK-293 Is Immoral, Goodbye Modern Medicine," Patheos: Through Catholic Lenses, January 28, 2021: https://www.patheos.com/blogs/throughcatholiclenses/2021/01/if-any-drug-tested-on-hek-293-is-immoral-goodbye-modern-medicine/ (Accessed on December 16, 2021). Unfortunately, he tries to argue the same point as the hospital in Little Rock. In his conclusion, Fr. Schneider, a Roman Catholic priest, rebukes those who selectively, as he puts it, reject abortion-related COVID-19 vaccines: "That is not an honest application of moral theology." Ironically, Fr. Schneider's unsubstantiated claims are rebuked, in turn, in Elizabeth Namati, "Yes, You Can Morally Object to a COVID Vax and Still Take Aspirin," The Stream, November 4, 2021: https://stream.org/yes-you-can-morally-object-to-a-covid-vax-and-still-take-aspirin/ (Accessed on December 16, 2021). Namati contends that only four of the prescription and over-the-counter medications that he cites owe their origin to aborted pre-born baby cell-lines! To be sure, the manufacturers of some of those products may have utilized aborted preborn baby cell lines for "quality control" many years later. If so, then my main argument below that we could disengage from those products gradually still would apply.

professing an absolute pacifist stance against all wars. Troup's cynical ploy, which other institutions have since invoked, entails a personal ad hominem presumption of moral inconsistency and dishonesty on the part of the hospital's employees. An overwhelming majority of opponents of COVID-19 vaccination on religious / moral grounds (yours truly included) are or were unaware of the omnipresence of the aborted preborn baby cell lines in medical practice and pharmaceuticals and are only now, thanks to the COVID-19 vaccine fiasco, coming to grips with the enormity of the problem. We are only beginning to develop a strategy for disengaging from the morally illicit vaccines and medicines "with all deliberate speed." That was the memorable phrase in the U.S. Supreme Court ruling against racial segregation in its Brown v. Board of Education decision in 1954. The highest court in the land did not expect every segregated school system in the United States to abolish the heinous practice and integrate immediately. Such a dramatic social change in institutions usually takes time to implement fully. The COVID-19 crisis is no different. In fact, the present challenge is more complex as conscientious Orthodox Christians and others now face a dramatic but necessary change in the rest of their lives.

Apart from the intrinsic evil of the COVID-19 vaccines themselves, one may profess a conscientious objection to the unprecedented draconian way that the COVID-19 vaccines were mandated upon a vulnerable population of thinking, conscientious employees. Moreover, this case is ripe for legal action by the employees involved, which could lead to the financial ruin of that hospital's corporation and other organizations that attempt to impose a false standard of moral "consistency."

Another challenge for faithful, conscientious Orthodox Christians in the present crisis is that public opinion on the issue is not on our side. The annual Gallup poll on moral issues dated May 18, 2021, revealed an increasing coarsening among most Americans on the issue of "stem cell research using human embryos." Fully 64% of those polled deem the practice "morally acceptable," while only 34% reject it as "morally wrong," compared to a 52% to 39% split on May 9, 2002. The same polls document a similar trend on the question of abortion. The American public has shifted from a 38% to 53% minority who regarded abortion as "morally acceptable" on May 9, 2002, to a very slim majority split of 47% to 46% on May 18, 2021.[56] Both trends are very lamentable, but it is odd that approximately 15% of those polled during the last nineteen years find nothing wrong with embryonic stem cell research while somehow opposing abortion. That kind of moral confusion also mars the pro-vaccine positions of many of the Orthodox leaders and faithful.

Faced with those dispiriting immoral practices and trends, a conscientious Orthodox Christian might surrender the moral argument out of a sense of futility, concede the impossibility of making a truly Orthodox moral choice, and decide to take one of the current COVID-19 vaccines along with any of the other medical / health vaccines, pharmaceuticals, or over-the-counter drugs connected to aborted preborn baby cell lines as the "lesser evil" and for the "greater good" of maintaining body health of oneself

---

56. Gallup, Inc., "Ratings of U.S. Moral Values": https://news.gallup.com/poll/1681/moral-issues.aspx (Accessed on December 16, 2021).

and others. But that would be a premature, foolish, and unworthy moral surrender.

First, there are genuinely moral alternatives to the abortion-related vaccines for a dozen notorious diseases. The Children of God for Life organization produced an excellent chart (updated as recently as January 2021) that indicates licit alternatives already available or in development for cystic fibrosis, Ebola, hemophilia, hepatitis A & B, hepatitis A & Typhoid, measles, mumps, Rubella, rabies, rheumatoid arthritis, shingles, and smallpox.[57] There is simply no excuse for anyone to resort to the old morally illicit vaccines for those afflictions.

Second, simply devoting personal time, diligence, and will-power might uncover morally licit equivalents to the pharmaceuticals and over-the-counter drugs on which we depend but are products of the Abortion-Doctor-Big Pharma Complex.

Third, if an Orthodox Christian concludes that he or she lacks the strength of will to refuse to take certain vaccines, pharmaceuticals, or over-the-counter drugs that are connected to aborted preborn baby cell lines, he might at least prod his conscience one more time and ask himself, "What is my soul worth? A dose of Tylenol?"

Fourth, it may mitigate the self-doubts and bolster the teetering moral sense within some of us to recall that a common counterargument in favor of taking any of the currently available COVID-19 vaccines—namely, "How can we selectively or even arbitrarily reject those vaccines on moral grounds, while still using so many other popular

---

57. https://cogforlife.org/wp-content/uploads/vaccineListOrigFormat.pdf (Accessed on December 16, 2021).

products with the same abortion industry pedigree?"—is essentially an *argument by deflection*. The logical fallacy is this: "Why can't we do this, since we already do that?" Applied to this case of COVID-19 vaccines, that appeal may seem prima facie to rise to a utilitarian philosophical argument for choosing immoral means to a good end for the most possible worthy beneficiaries. In truth, that reasoning is merely a sleight of hand that lumps all decisions together without due regard for the unique gravity and urgency of some crises and decisions over others. The present COVID-19 crisis demands our attention and our clear moral thinking and acting NOW! We can take care of the other seeming moral dilemmas and resolutions later.

Fifth, if an Orthodox Christian still concludes that he cannot avoid taking certain products that are connected to aborted preborn baby cell lines for other afflictions, he can still choose to draw the line here and now with the COVID-19 vaccine, especially in view of the dubious medical, political, and social pressures to "go along" with most of one's fellow Americans or the boss at work or the military commander or any of a host of persons in authority (including many Orthodox bishops!).

Without downplaying the 864,203 deaths in America out of 70,641,725 "confirmed" cases (a "case fatality rate" of 1.22% compared to approximately 30% for smallpox until it was eradicated in 1980) and the 5,592,266 "cumulative" deaths out of 349,641,119 "confirmed cases" around the globe (a "case fatality rate" of 1.60%) attributed so far to COVID-19,[58] I must observe that the COVID-19 crisis

---

58. See Centers for Disease Control (CDC, USA): https://covid.cdc.gov/covid-data-tracker/#trends_dailytrendscases; see and World Health Organization

is hardly the health apocalypse portrayed by many public officials and scientists (and, alas, Orthodox bishops) in the United States and elsewhere. Moreover, those case fatality rates have been slowly but steadily decreasing even during the most recent variants of COVID-19 that have led to new alarmist warnings, shutdowns, and other repressive mandates by various governments, including the United States. The continuing death toll of this crisis notwithstanding, Orthodox Christians ought to champion the divinely revealed truth that our life on earth is not all that God the Holy Trinity has given us. This life is a preparation for "the life of the world to come," as we recite in the Niceno-Constantinopolitan Creed. Are we so fearful of physical death that we would do anything to prolong our lives on this earth: compromise our consciences, justify all manner of evil actions, sacrifice others or willfully benefit from the unjust sacrifice—including murder—of others including preborn children? Have we forgotten since the last Pascha how St. John Chrysostom, Archbishop of Constantinople at the turn of the fourth century AD, exhorted us on that greatest feast of Church feasts, "Let no one fear death, for the death of the Savior has set us free!"

At the very least, therefore, let us make the COVID-19 crisis the line in the sand for a staunch, unyielding opposition to vaccines whose proponents and enforcers casually, cynically, and immorally exploit the abomination of the abortion of preborn babies. We might even follow the

---

(WHO): https://covid19.who.int/ (both accessed on January 24, 2022). The USA number of cases may be inflated by hospitals and others with a pecuniary interest in receiving federal dollars by designating COVID-19 as the *cause* of death when other factors were involved such as previous terminal illnesses or personal accidents.

example of tens of thousands of Greek citizens (most of them presumably Orthodox Christians) who staged massive public marches in Athens and other cities on July 14, 2021, to protest mandatory COVID-19 vaccinations.[59]   Or the reported dozen or so seminarians, "encouraged by at least one faculty member who is a priest," who launched an "anti-vaccination student movement" last summer in opposition to mandatory COVID-19 vaccines for all students at Holy Cross Greek Orthodox School of Theology in Brookline, Massachusetts, scheduled to begin in the Fall 2021 semester.[60] Alas, the Holy Cross administration cracked down hard on the resisters: several withdrew from the school and the others finally complied with the vaccine mandate before the 2021-2022 school year began.[61]   But there was at least a brief, shining moment of principled resistance at that institution.[62]

---

59. "Huge Demonstrations in Greece Against Mandatory Vaccinations!" *Helleniscope*, July 14, 2021: https://www.helleniscope.com/2021/07/14/huge-demonstrations-in-greece-against-mandatory-vaccination/ (Accessed on December 16, 2021).

60. "Anti-Vax Student Movement at Holy Cross School of Theology," *The National Herald*, July 20, 2021: https://www.thenationalherald.com/community_church_united_states/arthro/anti_vax_student_movement_at_holy_cross_school_of_theology-2927813/ That website, which I accessed on July 21, 2021, mysteriously no longer exists as of December 16, 2021. But *Helleniscope*, a website fiercely critical of the Greek Orthodox Archdiocese of America, also reported the story on July 21, 2021, under the title, "Student Anti-Vax Revolt in HCHC Exposes Once Again A Failing Leadership": https://www.helleniscope.com/2021/07/21/student-anti-vax-revolt-in-hchc-exposes-once-again-a-failing-leadership/ (Accessed on December 16, 2021, and still available on February 8, 2022).

61. Updated information on February 8, 2022, from a reliable source who requested anonymity.

62. Full disclosure: This turn of events is especially poignant for me. Before my graduation from Harvard Divinity School in 1978, I enrolled in five courses at nearby Holy Cross Greek Orthodox School of Theology taught by outstanding professors including Archimandrite (later Metropolitan) Maximos Aghiorgoussis, Protopresbyter Stanley Harakas, and Dr. Lewis Patsavos.

Our unbroken faith and hope in God the Holy Trinity and in the life in the world to come will sustain us in this present biological and moral trial. It will take that—as well as courage—to eschew tempting but immoral medical solutions to the COVID-19 virus, while waiting for a truly moral alternative.

May our Lord give us the strength to do so.

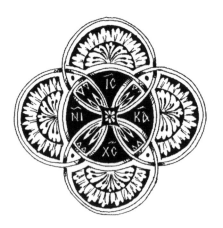

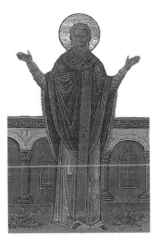

St. John the Faster,
Patriarch of Constantinople

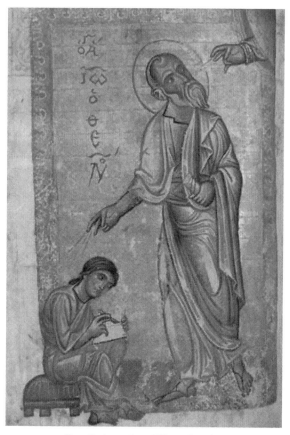

St. John the Theologian
"... discern the spirits..." I John 1:4:1-6

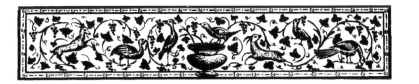

CHAPTER 8

The Demonic Methodology of the Coronavirus Narrative

Protopresbyter Peter Heers, D. Th.

From the appearance of the Coronavirus on the world stage, and the almost immediate debut of the Covid-19 pandemic narrative, the tell-tale signs of a demonic methodology were apparent: fear, anxiety, confusion, inconsistency and contradiction, coercion, threats, censorship, misinformation, half-truths and lies. This was a spiritual challenge of the greatest magnitude. The way in which the new crisis was presented and confronted revealed—or should have revealed—to all watchful Orthodox Christians, the origins and nature of the "crisis." What we were confronting was no simple "health matter" for which the Church must listen obediently to "the experts" and meekly obey the governments which these experts were guiding. Rather, the demonic methodology of the coronavirus narrative put us all on notice that beyond the virus and the threat it posed to bodily health, the Church was confronting a grave and terrible spirit of delusion and deception, coercion, and manipulation.

The Discernment of Spirits

For those who balk at such a decisive affirmation of the demonic nature of the crisis, it is necessary for them to recall that the discernment of spirits belongs to the Church in Her saints and the holy fathers of the Church, as well as to those who follow their life and teachings closely. Indeed, the difference between Orthodoxy and heterodoxy is most apparent in that the Orthodox Church (in Her saints) can discern the spirits. Discernment of the methods of the fallen spirits is so essential that it is a requirement for the proper formation of Christology and Ecclesiology. As the Evangelist John writes, "For this purpose the Son of God was manifested, that he might destroy the works of the devil" (1 John 3:8).

It would not be an exaggeration to state that, alongside philanthropy and evangelical preaching, that which the Church has to offer to all good-willed truth-seekers is Her prophetic voice of truth, rightly discerning the spirits and exposing to the light the machinations of the enemy, according to the Apostle Paul:

> [H]ave no fellowship with the unfruitful works of darkness, but rather reprove them. For it is a shame even to speak of those things which are done of them in secret. But all things that are reproved are made manifest by the light: for whatsoever doth make manifest is light. (Ephesians 5:11-13).

Therefore, without a doubt the role of the Church in the current darkness brought about by the Covid-19 pandemic narrative is to provide a spiritual analysis of events and to navigate the faithful through the challenges and hard decisions they are facing by such menaces as church closures, innovations in worship and vaccine mandates.[1]

Caesaropapism: The Subordination of Clergy to Secular Power

Tragically, instead of offering the prophetic voice and stance of the Saints, much of the current leadership of the Church has, when not running ahead of tyrannical governmental overreach, passively acquiesced to it. Instead of identifying secularism, the very spirit of Antichrist, as animating and guiding State-sponsored church closures (even as child-murder factories remained open), some church leaders justified the intrusions as benevolent and philanthropic. Most observers were stunned at the ease by which Caesar, during the manufactured storm,[2] was given

---

1. The great Saint of Mt. Athos, universally venerated, Elder Paisios, spoke prophetically about the current vaccine mandates (compulsory vaccination did not exist in Greece in the 1980s): "Now a vaccine has been developed to combat a new disease, which will be obligatory, and those taking it will be marked" (*Spiritual Counsels II: Spiritual Awakening*, page 204, Holy Monastery of St. John the Theologian, Souroti, Thessaloniki, December 2008).

2. The blessed Elder Savvas Achilleos (+2016), also spoke about a future flu and vaccine. In his lifetime, some clergy claimed that Elder Savvas was deceived and a "conspiracy theorist." He was also persecuted by his own bishop. The following was taken from a homily he gave on October 11, 2007: "They are warning us that the flu is coming. How do they know this? How do they know? Tell me, how? It is because they themselves will manufacture it and release it. This will not be a common epidemic form of the flu, but a flu that will come when they themselves will bring it upon the world. A manufactured disease right from the United States of America. What causes this new disease which looks like the common flu? It is caused by a pathogenic mycoplasma…It will be transmitted through an anti-flu vaccine. This is the point where we must be careful. The world will feel the need to receive the anti-flu shot, yet this vaccine will contain a cruel illness in and of itself and will not contain anything that will prevent people from contracting the virus. It is highly recommended to not proceed to any vaccination." How do our contemporary clergy ignore this most obvious prophetic utterance?

the helm to steer the ship of the Church into the "peaceful harbor" of the non-essentials of society—in truth not a harbor at all but a ship-graveyard.

Christ's sheep, kept away from the sheepfold by order of the wolves of this world, all, of course, "for their protection," were nevertheless exposed to a most deadly plague. Swooping down upon the Christian people was the scourge of secularism. Unprecedented and unconscionable were the closing of the Holy Temples of God, the abandoning of the faithful and the denial of the medicine of immortality. Furthermore, flagrantly opposed to the freedom Orthodox Christians have—who are not only created in the Image of God but also being restored to His Likeness—stood those hierarchs who either sought to pressure clergy and faithful to receive vaccines or denied them recourse to the Church for vaccine exemptions. The utter subjection of some hierarchs to the anti-ecclesial agenda of many governments will undoubtedly be commemorated by faithful church historians as one of the most shameful periods of Church history, reminiscent of Metropolitan Sergius of Moscow's "Declaration" in 1927, which pledged complete loyalty—and more—to the Soviet Union under the notorious Communist dictator Josef Stalin.[3]

---

3. This sentence captures best the extent of the collaboration of the Russian Orthodox Church with the vicious Soviet regime: "We want to be Orthodox and at the same time to be conscious of the Soviet Union as our civil motherland, whose joys and successes are our joys and successes and whose failures, failures. Any blow directed at the Union, be it a war, a boycott, a public calamity or just a treacherous murder, like one in Warsaw, is recognized as a blow aimed at us. While remaining Orthodox, we remember our duty to be citizens of the Union 'not only out of fear, but also for conscience's sake,' as the Apostle teaches us (Romans XIII, 5)." For an English translation of that official statement of the Russian Orthodox Church see https://www.rocorstudies.org/2017/06/09/3098/.

The Temple of Thy Glory—a Common Place?

Standing in the temple of thy glory, we think
ourselves to stand in Heaven, O Theotokos
— Lenten Matins

Not long after the outset of the "pandemic" we heard of cases where bishops were ordering the closure of the churches ahead of any state mandates, all in the name of the bodily health of the people. The fear was that the faithful would become ill in the Temple, and the basis given for closures was the evangelical command to love our neighbor: "Thou shalt love thy neighbour as thyself" (Matt. 22:39). That is, since those bishops regarded the Temple of God is a place like any other with respect to illness and death, love of neighbor necessitated closing it down.

Is this, however, the witness of the Holy Fathers regarding the Holy Temple? Is it possible to shut down the churches, keep people from the Fount of Incorruption, and yet do this out of love for our neighbor? Do we have any precedent for this not only in Church history (one can always find exceptions) but in the examples and lives of the Holy Fathers whom we follow? What do our Holy Fathers and Saints say about the Temple of God and our stance within it? St. John of Kronstadt, that great righteous one and man of prayer, emphasized:

> "Truly the church is Heaven upon earth; for where the throne of God is, where the awful sacraments are celebrated, where the angels serve together with men, ceaselessly glorifying the Almighty, there is

truly Heaven.[4] And so let us enter into the house of God with the fear of God, with a pure heart, **laying aside all vices and every worldly care, and let us stand in it with faith and reverence**, with understanding attention, **with love and peace in our hearts**, so that we may come away renewed, as though made Heavenly; so that we may **live in the holiness natural to Heaven, not bound by worldly desires and pleasures.**"[5]

Can one stand in the Temple with reverence, as in Heaven, laying aside all worldly care, when inundated with anxiety-ridden measures and divisive liturgical innovations? Does this reverent stance allow any room for the innovations we have seen introduced into the Divine Services over the past two years: roping off of Holy Icons, masking, social distancing, limiting of participation and banning of the kiss of peace, multiple lavidas (spoons) and their cleansing with alcohol, and other such practices borrowed from the graceless, rationalist, worldly-minded, who live outside of the Body of Christ?

Or, what about this understanding and stance vis-a-vis the Holy Temple and the holy things within, expressed by the great dogmatic theologian and confessor of the Faith, St. Justin Popovich? Can it be reconciled with the innovations?

Every Holy Temple is a piece of heaven on the earth. And **when you are in the Temple you are already found to be in heaven**. So, when the earth

---

4. Boldface added here and elsewhere in this chapter for emphasis.

5. St. John of Kronstadt, My life in Christ excerpt in Spiritual Counsels of Father John of Kronstadt, ed. by W. J. Grisbrooke. N.Y.: SVS Press, 1967.

causes you anguish with its hell, run to the Temple, enter in and **you are in paradise**! And if the people are tormenting you with their evil intentions, run and take refuge in the Temple and kneel before God and He will take you under His sweet and all-powerful protection. If, once again, it happens that a whole host of demons are pouncing upon you again, run to the Temple, amidst the Angels, **for the Temple is always full of Angels**, and the Angels of God will **protect you from all of the demons of the world, and they will be rendered powerless to do you harm**.[6]

Can one take refuge in the Temple as in paradise when the hell of anxiety and fear enter the Holy Temple by way of the innovations? Or can we still be sure that demonic machinations are rendered powerless when we ourselves are carrying within us the fear of death and trust in fallen men and their "salvation" into the Temple? Shall we blame God for our giving of "rights" to the enemy and the possible consequences we may bring upon ourselves by our lack of trust in His protection?

Or can this ancient witness to the meaning and nature of the Divine Liturgy by St. Germanos of Constantinople be reconciled with the stance taken when conducting the innovations?

The church is **the temple of God, a holy place**, a house of prayer, the assembly of the people, the body of Christ. The church is **an earthly heaven in**

---

6. St. Justin Popovoch, from "Velka Gospojina, 1963," "Na Bogocovecanskom Putu."

which the supercelestial God dwells and walks about. The Church is **heaven on earth, where God lives and dwells**, Who is higher than heaven. . . It calls to mind the crucifixion, the burial and the resurrection of Christ, it is more glorious than the Tabernacle of the Covenant. . . It was prefigured in the patriarchs, founded on the apostles . . . it was foretold by the prophets, adorned by the hierarchs, sanctified by the martyrs, and its altar is founded on their holy relics. . . The church is **a divine house** where the mysterious and life-giving sacrifice takes place, where there is the inner sanctuary, the holy cave, the sepulchre, the soul-saving and **life-giving food**, where you will find the pearls of the divine doctrines which the Lord taught His disciples.[7]

The rationalist Christian will dismiss all the above as pious expressions void of any practical, "scientific" importance for "policy-making" in the age of Covidism. So be it. For the Orthodox Christian, who lives by faith, the faith of the Lord Jesus Christ, the all-powerful protection of God promised to His faithful children is not limited to a part of man, his soul, but extends to the whole man—by the Grace of that Man Who assumed our nature, which now sits at the right of the Father. For the Orthodox Christian, to stand with faith and reverence and to enter the love and peace of the Lord in His Temple is incompatible with, if not opposed to, the stance of the "covidists" and their "priestly class" of expert scientists, which see the Temple as another supermarket, only selling "religion."

---

7. St. Germanus of Constantinople, *On the Divine Liturgy*. Trans. Paul Meyendorff. Crestwood, NY, 1984.

It is impossible to reconcile the stance of the rationalists with that of the Saints, who implicitly trust the Lord always, but most especially while in the embrace of His Grace in His Temple. Consider the enlightening words of the renowned, ever-memorable elder of Simonopetra Monastery on Mt. Athos, Archimandrite Aimilianos, as he calls the faithful to enter deeply into the ethos and mindset of the Church in the Temple:

> "Where is Christ? Here and everywhere! Above all, Christ, the second person of the Holy Trinity, is seated within the Holy of Holies, at the right hand of the heavenly Father. So **don't think that when we go to church, we are simply entering and exiting an ordinary building. Instead, we go up to, and make our entrance into, the Holy of Holies, into the heavens themselves**. As we open the curtain of the Royal Doors, and Christ is present in the Holy Chalice, so do we sinners open the doors of heaven and enter! . . . . When we enter church, then, we are traversing the distance from earth to heaven. We pass beyond the stars, we leave the angels below us, and **we rise up to the heights of the Holy Trinity. This is the mystery of our Church**... The same mystery is enacted here, outside the space of the sanctuary. In front of us we see various images, above us are the lamps, each hanging next to the other. But that's wrong. **These too are a part of the mystery. We are not here. We are up there, together with the assemblies of the Saints, together with the ranks of the angels**, with the six-winged Seraphim—whose swift movements teach

us to hasten day and night to Christ—together with the cherubim of many eyes, so that our own eyes can become accustomed to seeing Christ. This is a sacrament. This is what a "Mystery" of the Church means . . . So, **we have come to church, to the Liturgy! Let nothing disturb the tranquility of your soul. God is present. Wherever we look, God is before us! If we don't see Him, this doesn't mean He isn't there, but only that our eyes are not used to seeing him**. At the end of the Divine Liturgy, we proclaim, 'We have seen the true light.' Our hearts have seen it. We have felt it deep within our life."[8]

When we enter the Temple, where God is present, where "nothing must disturb the tranquility of the soul," we depart from this earth and enter heaven, where there is no sighing or sorrow or pain, but life everlasting. Orthodox Christians do not wait to enter paradise after death; they enter paradise now, in this present life, or not at all. There is no return (repentance) to paradise after death, when man is not whole, when he is not proper man.[9] It is "another gospel" that heretics preach and that supposes paradise to be limited to certain bodiless angels and bodiless men and not brought into this world in the Body of Christ, in the Temple of His glory.

---

8. "Our Church Attendance: Reflections on the Divine Liturgy of St. James" in *The Church at Prayer*.

9. St. John of Damascus, restating the patristic view, as expressed, for example by St. Maximus the Confessor, writes that there can be no repentance for demons after their fall, just as there can be none after death for man. Cf. John of Damascus, On the Orthodox Faith 17 (= II.3); ed. P. Bonifatius Kotter, *Die Schriften des Johannes von Damaskos* (Berlin: De Gruyter, 1969-88), vol. 2, 46, trans. FOC 37, 206.

And it is "another gospel," preached by those whose "eyes are not used to seeing Christ" in the paradise of the Temple and whose feet are still mired in the "dust of the ground" and whose nostrils do not regularly inhale the "breath of life," that supposes the Temple of Life to be a common place governed by the laws of the fallen world, not overcoming, but succumbing entirely to the "laws of nature." To them St. Athanasius speaks and says, "Seek not how this is so, for where God wills the order of nature is overcome."[10]

In the Orthodox Church, which is the Body of Christ, the Temple of God, the consecrated, "baptized" Temple where the Holy Spirit descends as on Pentecost and fills all with Light and transforms men into God-men by Grace, where not only the bread and wine but the faithful themselves are changed into the Body of Christ, it is not only the Holy Communion which is sanctified, so as to make it and all that touches it (i.e., the holy *lavida*, or spoon) impossible to be a communicant and carrier of sin, death and disease (which are the result of the fall away from Life), since He is Life, a Fire which burns away all impurity, but indeed all that which is holy and set apart by God because God dwells therein—such as the Holy Icons, the Holy Relics, the Holy Antidoron (blessed bread), and even the hand of the priest, who is the type and in the place of Christ and whose hands touch the Immaculate Body, or even the Holy Embrace shared by the priest and faithful (when we say "Christ is in our midst; He

---

10. St. Athanasius the Great, *Homily on the Nativity of Christ*: "I behold a strange mystery: instead of the sun, the sun of righteousness contained ineffably in the Virgin. Seek not how this is so, for where God wills the order of nature is overcome. It was His will, He had the power to do so, and thus He came down and saved us." https://www.oca.org/news/headline-news/metropolitan-tik-hons-nativity-message-released.

is and ever shall be!")—that is sanctified and thus free of
corruption, which is a fruit of the fallen world.

Therefore, in the Orthodox Church—whether or not
all understand this or act upon it, or even if nearly all are
ignorant of it and fall away from it—it is at least faithlessness,
if not worse (God forbid!), blasphemy, to treat the Holy
Things of the Holy Temple—consecrated and set apart by
and in God—as common, that is, as we would and do in the
supermarket, bank or post office. Therefore, it is a fall away
from this self-understanding, this experience of God's Grace,
this way of being in Christ, to bring into the Holy Temple, as
into a common place, masks, gloves, multiple spoons (for fear
of communicating viruses) and the like. In the Temple of
God, consecrated and sanctified by and to God, the Church
of Christ has nothing to fear (fear is of the evil one), for the
members of the Body are in the Temple of the Body, in the
embrace of the Father, in the communion of the Holy Spirit.

The Two Greatest and Inseparable Commandments

Like that snake of old which slithered into the garden,
the fear of disease and death crept into the paradise of the
Temple of God. This devilish fear was not only behind
the overcoming of the order of the Church, in deference
to the "order of [fallen] nature," it was likewise behind the
cessation of the offering of the Sacrifice to the faithful. Thus,
the closure of the churches had not only an immediate and
detrimental impact on the spiritual life of the members of
the Body, by depriving them of the nourishment of prayer
and the Mystery of Mysteries; it deprived the world of that

without which it would soon cease to be, and, consequently, it gave wide berth to demons to deceive. The effect was immediate and extensive: the devil walked "naked" through life and society, inspiring "evil men and seducers" to wax "worse and worse, deceiving, and being deceived" (2 Tim. 3:13). With the docile approval of the shepherds, the enemy took advantage of the scattering of the sheep and their spiritual starvation and pounded them with relentless, brain-numbing fearmongering, convincing many that the "miraculous" solution promised was the "shot from God" and the only "light at the end of the tunnel."

The tragic image of scattered sheep and scared shepherds should not have come as a great surprise to a watchful observer. Preceding this division was another, that of the horizontal and vertical bars of Christ's Greatest Commandment: the inseparable love for God and for man.

The Lord commanded all His disciples:

> "Thou shalt love the Lord thy God with all thy heart, and with all thy soul, and with all thy mind. This is the first and great commandment. And the second *is* like unto it, Thou shalt love thy neighbour as thyself. On these two commandments hang all the law and the prophets" (Matthew 22: 37-40).

The churches were closed, the Sacrifice inaccessible, the congregation disassembled, His commandments set aside, all in the name of loving one's neighbor. The Church had descended "out of love" to the social plane. Yet, the two commandments are as one and the order in which they were given is immutable. When the second is placed first or made autonomous, the first is not simply undermined, it is undone, set aside. True love of neighbor—such as seeking to shield him from illness—*presupposes* the transfiguring, all-embracing love of God. Well established in the "first love" of God (Rev. 2:4), man is then truly able to love His neighbor. Absent this greater commandment, his love is not true, not transformative, not salvific. Such love, lacking in divine ("vertical") / human ("horizontal") synergy is not *theanthropic, and not crucified.* Such love is "of this world" and makes the Church take on the color of "another gospel," the new "social gospel" of humanism and other sundry 'isms' of our latter days, first of which is secularism, the spirit of Antichrist.

The Only Hospital of the Whole Man Closed by Order of the Physicians

As the hospitals of the body were said to be overrun, the only hospital of the soul was closed. The tragedy of the closing of the churches is not at all limited to the disorder it introduced into the Temple or into the hierarchy of loves, or into our souls as a result. The tragedy is compounded by the fatal irony of the only true physicians of souls and bodies—the clergy—boarding up their practice (churches) just as their services were being universally sought—and this mockingly in the name of "love" and "humility," since (it was assumed to be obvious) the "pandemic" was only a "medical issue" for which "experts" must be consulted and uncritically heeded. Unless, that is, you trusted the "wrong" experts, who stood opposed to the narrative and the newfangled vaccines; then you were guilty of being "proud" and "dangerously reckless," even akin to—brace yourself—a schismatic, a Nazi, or even an "antichrist"!

Truly, blind obedience to the narrative led churchmen into desperate straits, for what could be more tragic than the only hospital of souls and bodies closing its doors just as a spiritual plague of unprecedented dissimulation hit? When a doctor hangs up his stethoscope during an epidemic and goes on vacation, his conscience must accuse him and his empty heart refuse him joy. But the spiritual doctor? What of his conscience? How is it that it was not more sensitive to his patients, even as they knocked on his door for the saving Mysteries and instead of the prayer of forgiveness, he read them Caesar's latest directive "for their own good." Where is the love of neighbor here? Absent, of course, along with the fear of God. Not surprisingly, the world and worldly hailed them, their own, as "lovers of humanity," while those opposed to declaring spiritual bankruptcy and shuttering church doors were compared to heretical snake handlers.

In past times, the Church not only did not close its doors to the needy, demon-ridden world—let alone to Her own members—she flung them open and marched out into the streets wielding Her weapons of peace and healing. Repeatedly the Holy relics and wonderworking icons of God sanctified creation and drove out demonically inflicted disease, and "the order of nature" was overcome as the Lord so willed in response to the pleas of those who walked "by the faith of the Son of God" (Gal. 2:20). The same power of trust which provided God occasion to extinguish the flames which bore down on the Monastery of Saint David in Evia, Greece, in the summer of 2021 could and should have been on display in countless parishes and dioceses worldwide for the entirety of the "pandemic." That in the context of Covid-19 Christ was defamed by His own disciples and deprived of the opportunity to pronounce "according to your faith, be it done to you" is not easily explained and must not be quickly dismissed. It must be attributed to something unique and unprecedented—the display of demonic delusion during the unfolding of the Covid fear and coercion narrative.

The Demonic Methodology of the Coronavirus Narrative

In the diabolical "ethics" of this world, the end alone justifies the means. In the heavenly ethos of the saints, *good is not good, if not done in a good way.*[11] This necessarily narrows matters, making the Christian way overly "impractical" for the worldly minded. However, for the "violent man" of the Gospel (Matt. 11:12) this basic patristic principle still acts as a compass to navigate a way through the thick clouds of confusion, half-truths, lies and governmental propaganda, to remain Orthodox, even if we do not have—or *do* have—a higher level degree in medicine, science or "bioethics."

Our Lord said that "I am the way, the truth, and the life: no man cometh unto the Father, but by me" (John 14:6). Those three are inseparable, such that when (not if) we are discerning the spirits (1 John 4: 1-5) of this world (the ideas, currents, and spiritual and intellectual movements in the world) we must assess their origins and aims based on not only the truth but also the way and the life. The way we do something reveals as much about its origins and aims as whether it is true. The life a spirit (idea or claim) inspires or contributes to, the fruit it produces (Matt. 7:16-20), tells us as much about its nature (being of God or of the

---

11. "τό καλόν οὐκ ἔστι καλόν, ἐάν μή καλῶς γένηται". See St. Ephraim the Syrian (*Works*, 106.406) and St. John of Damascus (*Exposition on Faith*, 25:87).

enemy) as does the truth of its claims or the way in which it is being employed. In this way of discerning things, among others, our Lord has given all—irrespective of their rational intellect's formation (or disformation) in the education centers of this world—the means to be watchful and to avoid the deceit of the enemy. It was, lest we forget, to fishermen that He revealed the Mysteries of the Kingdom, not the highly educated, and thus the tools He gives His disciples for navigating their spiritual way are both simple and accessible to the humble and profound and inaccessible to the proud.

With this spiritual approach, then, the demonic methodology of the coronavirus narrative is not hard to spot. It violates a foundational spiritual law, *good is not good, if not done in a good way*, and does so in a flagrant manner. Nevertheless, serious churchmen refuse to acknowledge this or the consequences of it. As we said from the outset, the way in which the "pandemic" narrative was presented and confronted, and the fruit of its implementation—the life we led and are leading—reeked of the demonic, plunging men into fear, anxiety, and confusion, medical professionals into inconsistency and contradiction, and governmental officers into coercion, threats, censorship, misinformation, half-truths and lies.

Amazingly, in the midst of this demonic state of things we are told by some churchmen that God has brought forth a "miracle," a God-sent solution which only a fool would reject: a novel gene-tweaking technology baptized as a "vaccine," which does not (they always neglect to note) prevent contraction or transmission of the virus.[12] Yet worse, in terms of spiritual delusion, and in the face of the most

---

12. See footnote #1 above.

serious ethical concerns arising from the employment of cell lines derived from murdered and dismembered unborn babies, we hear professors and clergymen stunningly accept as *fait accompli* the light-hearted abandonment of the patristic axiom and adoption of a utilitarian approach to the taking of these "vaccines"—an approach so antithetical to the narrow Way of the Lord.

Fear of Death is Bondage, Fear of God, Freedom

The fear of death is a most powerful force, one that, it appears, has been able to draw Orthodox Christians into justifying Godless means for supposedly "good ends." This is an unjustified supposition, In the case of these novel gene technologies even a utilitarian ethic is hardly warranted, since it is not yet apparent that the greatest good has come about for the greatest number of people. What is already apparent, at least, is that for the greatest part of humanity a gross and health-compromising dependency upon endless, if also feeble, booster shots has been secured, along with a gross and wealth-enhancing dependency upon (and in favor of) Big Pharma. In both respects, the whole of humanity has been placed within a two-fold bondage—physical and financial—and the paradigm of Godless utilitarians allows for no escape.

However, before this external enslavement there was a spiritual enslavement. If we consider the matter from the more important and higher perspective, the spiritual, a three-fold bondage becomes apparent. The fear of death has led many to trade in not just his physical and financial freedom for the "security" of a Big Pharma managed "vax-plan" and Big Government socialist health-control plan.

The fear of death has led many today to cease living truly and truly living at all. Even sincere Orthodox Christians are fearfully trampling upon their consciences as they receive what they believe to be a *pharmakon* (with the original Greek meaning poison), for the sake of securing, for themselves and their family, "an existence" which they know is not true life. Only when one lives for and in God, *for and in the Truth*, does "[he] have life," and "have it more abundantly" (John 10:10). When the billion-dollar revenue generating, gene-tweaking technology is being manipulatively pushed through totalitarian mandates upon innocent and unaffected five-year-olds the world over, that should be *more* than enough for all to understand the demonic origins and aims of the coronavirus narrative.

Of course, this is no mere health matter, for there *is* no *mere* health matter. Such a thing emphatically does not exist, nor ever could. The arena of the spiritual battle touches every aspect of our life, and everyone, whether he likes it or knows it, is standing, fighting, or falling, in the spiritual stadium of this life. We are embodied spiritual beings, so the enemy of our salvation, aping and inverting Christ and His disciples (1 Cor. 9:22), uses *everything* for our damnation. As ecclesiastical history teaches us, Lucifer has regularly found useful servants to hear his call and implement his schemes. The summons today for "blind obedience" to medical, scientific, or even ecclesiastical "experts" by Orthodox Christians, let alone clergy, succeeds only in revealing the callers' spiritual blindness as to the signs of the times and stage of the ever-evolving apostasy.

Having "put on Christ" in Baptism in the Church, however, the Orthodox Christian has been delivered from the bondage and blindness brought about through the "fear of death" (Heb. 2:15). This Freedom (John 8:32), which is given to those who have loved the Truth (2 Thess. 2:10), the criterion of those who will be saved in the last days, is the priceless treasure for which he will sell everything (Matt. 13:44-46) and for which every Truth-seeker will seek him out as a savior who leads to the One Savior. These "free in Christ" and God-fearing will gladly suffer everything, even death (whether by God's allowance or good will), to retain the priceless Truth. They will stand opposed to the coronavirus narrative and its "one-way out" vaccine "final solution," gladly suffering mockery, heckling, and depersonalization as egotistical "anti-vaxers" guilty of "fratricide." Few will understand this stance as an extension and expression of the hope that is in the Truth-lover. But, as the Apostle Peter wrote,

> "If ye suffer for righteousness' sake, happy are ye: and be not afraid of their terror, neither be troubled; But sanctify the Lord God in your hearts: and be ready always to give an answer to every man that asketh you a reason of the hope that is in you with meekness and fear: Having a good conscience; that, whereas they speak evil of you, as of evildoers, they may be ashamed that falsely accuse your good conversation in Christ" (1 Peter 3: 14-16).

Straight ahead we can most assuredly expect tribulation, but we are cheerful for we know that the Lord has overcome the world (John 16:33). This joy of living in the Truth—and enduring persecution for it—will be a sign (Luke 2:34) of the true Christian. The capitulation to the mantra of fear-mongers who bring "peace and security" (1 Thess. 5:3) will reveal the "new Christians." These are, as Fr. Seraphim Rose has written, those men,

> who the increasingly menacing powers of the world seduce to compromise with the obvious and union with the forces of the worldly. It would be insanity, surely to do anything else, so speak the worldly. The true Christian is, in the eyes of the world, insane. He trusts in a God who can and will preserve him in the midst of the most painful torture and death…What the Roman Caesars attempted to accomplish with their limited means, the impersonal powers of the world today attempt with much more impressive means of modern technology. Both must fail when confronted with a faith that truly reaches out beyond this world. And such faith the Christian has if he remains true to Christ.[13]

Remaining Fearless for Christ before the Face of Antichrist

In the age of Antichrist, as we are daily swimming in a sea of lies and propaganda, remaining true to Christ will require a true crucifixion of the intellect and will. For, even as the world seeks to "move heaven and earth" to avoid suffering and death, "the Christian accepts them, and indeed welcomes them. For he knows that without such trials, there is no progress in the spiritual life."[14] Indeed, in the face of the march toward a "new humanity" and the attempt at a

---

13. Eugene Rose, "Christian Realism and Worldly Idealism."

14. Ibid.

technological transcendence of the effects of the Fall, the Christian, with fear of God and faith and love,

> expects from life no more, nor less, than the crucifixion his Lord endured. The inevitable end of the world is something that the worldly dread, so they must somehow realize, whether they acknowledge it or not, that this is the final mockery of all their comfortable faith. But the Christian has no consolation in the worldly superstition of the indefinite future, for he knows the last days are indeed at hand.[15]

This eschatological stance indicates a true Christian and sets him on a collision course with the world and its "new humanism" and "social gospel," which seeks not the heavenly Kingdom of the Church but a "new world order" and "great reset"—the same lie of the serpent repackaged, to become gods without God, to set up a utopia among the ruins of our humanity.

We are coming full circle: the Church is surrounded again by an antagonistic, neo-pagan society that hates Christ and Christians, but this time with unprecedented vigor. As we face the continued spread of the spiritual plague of secularism, of which covidism is a by-product, we would do well to remember how the early Christians lived and died during times of an actual pandemic and to imitate their fearlessness of death and faith in Christ.

St. Dionysius of Alexandria describes how the Christians and pagans encountered the scourge:

> The most of our brethren were unsparing in their exceeding love and brotherly *kindness. They held fast to*

---

15. Ibid.

each other and visited the sick fearlessly, and ministered to them
continually, serving them in Christ. And they died with
them most joyfully, taking the affliction of others, and
drawing the sickness from their neighbors to themselves
and willingly receiving their pains. And many who cared
for the sick and gave strength to others died themselves
having transferred to themselves their death. And the
popular saying which always seems a mere expression
of courtesy, they then made real in action, taking their
departure as the others' 'offscouring.'

"Truly the best of our brethren departed from life
in this manner, including some presbyters and deacons
and those of the people who had the highest reputation;
so that this form of death, through the great piety and
strong faith it exhibited, seemed to lack nothing of
martyrdom.

"And they took the bodies of the saints in their
open hands and in their bosoms, and closed their eyes
and their mouths; and they bore them away on their
shoulders and laid them out; and they clung to them
and embraced them; and they prepared them suitably
with washings and garments. And after a little they
received like treatment themselves, for the survivors
were continually following those who had gone before
them.

"But with the heathen everything was quite
otherwise. They deserted those who began to be sick,
and fled from their dearest friends. And they cast
them out into the streets when they were half dead,
and left the dead like refuse, unburied. They shunned
any participation or fellowship with death; which yet,

with all their precautions, it was not easy for them to escape."[16]

Without God, there is no hope; without God, no one escapes this life alive. The only questions that truly matter are these: How will we live and how will we die? The two are inseparable. Death is the fruit of our life, the quintessential moment for each person. Will we imitate Christ and the Saints, and follow the Holy Fathers? Will we love Christ and overcome fear?

Those are the two questions that must frame everything we ponder and decide to do in the present crisis. The trials and tests to date, deceptions and delusions, church closures and vaccine mandates, are just the beginning of the pangs that are coming upon the world. Let them be a bell, to wake us up from our slumber and set us out on the narrow path with redoubled zeal, on *the path of repentance* for indifference to Truth, for embracing a utilitarian ethic, for ignoring the hierarchy of love, for trampling upon our conscience, for exchanging confession of faith for safety and freedom for job security, for trusting in the "experts" of the world over the Creator of the world, and for succumbing to the demonic methodology of the narrative. Let us strengthen ourselves to remain committed to Christ before the rise of the spirit of Antichrist and the loss of not only our comfort and goods, but even our own life. Then the truth of our faith will be apparent, the kingdom of God will be revealed to all, the demonic methodology of the enemy will be overcome in us, and Christ will be glorified.

---

16. Eusebius, *Ecclesiastical History*, Book VII, Chapter 22: 7-10.

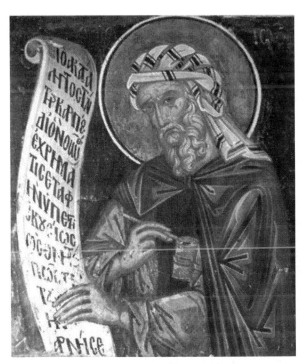

St. John of Damascus

NOTES ON
CONTRIBUTORS

Metropolitan Jonah (James Paffhausen) was born in Chicago and grew up in the San Diego area. He was raised Episcopalian and found Orthodoxy at university and converted at the age of 19. After graduating from the University of California, Santa Cruz, with a B.A. in Anthropology, he completed the degrees of Master of Divinity and Master of Theology in Dogmatics at St Vladimir's Orthodox Theological Seminary in Crestwood, New York. He pursued doctoral studies in Berkeley, CA, before moving to Russia, where he joined Valaam Monastery and remained from two years. Metropolitan Jonah returned to the United States in 1993 and was ordained the following year to the Diaconate and Priesthood in the Orthodox Church in America (OCA). He worked to establish mission churches in the USA; in 1996 he established the Monastery of St John of San Francisco in Point Reyes Station, later Manton, CA. In 2008 he was elected the Auxiliary to Archbishop Dmitri of Dallas (OCA). Only eleven days later Bishop Jonah was elected as Metropolitan, Primate, of the Orthodox Church in America. He served in that capacity for almost four years. In 2015 Metropolitan Jonah was received as the retired OCA Primate by the Russian Orthodox Church Outside of Russia (ROCOR). In 2017 he accepted an assignment as Rector of St Herman of Alaska Church, Stafford, Virginia (ROCOR). In 2020, he established the Monastery of St. Demetrios in Spotsylvania, Virginia, and serves as spiritual father and abbot. Metropolitan Jonah continues to lecture and write for publication, teach various classes in person and online, produce videos, and conduct retreats.

Archpriest Alexander F. C. Webster, Ph.D., retired in August 2019 as Dean and Professor of Moral Theology Emeritus at Holy Trinity Orthodox Seminary in Jordanville, New York. He also retired in June 2010 as a U.S. Army chaplain in the rank of Colonel after a quarter century of service in uniform, his last five years back on active duty primarily to conduct twelve periodic visits to the American and Coalition troops of Eastern Orthodox Christian faith in the combat areas of Afghanistan and Iraq, as well as Kuwait and Qatar. Archpriest Alexander holds academic degrees in History from the University of Pennsylvania (A.B., 1972), History & Education from Columbia University (M.A., 1975), Theology from Harvard University Divinity School (M.T.S.,1977), and Religion / Social Ethics from the University of Pittsburgh (Ph.D., 1988). In addition to 50 scholarly articles and book chapters, as well as more than 100 op-ed articles and interviews in newspapers, magazines, and online, he is the author of four books on religious ethical themes and co-editor of another. Following ordination to the Holy Priesthood in September 1982, he served for a total of 26 years as rector of Orthodox parishes in Clairton, PA, Falls Church, VA, and Stafford, VA. Currently adjunct professor of Religious Studies at George Mason University, Archpriest Alexander has also taught at eleven institutions of higher education including George Washington University, Virginia Theological Seminary, and the University of Maryland University College in Okinawa, Japan. He has been married for 49 years to Matushka Kathleen, and they are blessed with four children and three grandchildren.

Protopresbyter Peter A. Heers, D.Th. was born in Dallas, Texas and grew up near San Francisco. The son of an Anglican priest, in 1992 his parents and much of his father's parish converted to the Orthodox Church. In 1996 he came to Thessaloniki, Greece, in order to visit Mt. Athos, returning again in 1998 to begin the Theological School of the University of Thessaloniki. He lived in the area for 19 years, where he married a Thessaloniki native (and blessed with 5 children). He was ordained to the diaconate and priesthood in 2003, in the Diocese of Kastoria. Fr. Peter has undergraduate, masters and doctoral degrees in Dogmatic Theology from the Theological School of the University of Thessalonica, all completed under the tutelage of Professor Demetrios Tselingides. He was the rector and spiritual father of the parish of the Holy Prophet Elias in Petrokerasa, a small village in the mountains outside of Thessalonica, Greece, from 2006 until 2017. In 2014 he was made Protopresbyteros and Spiritual Father of the Diocese of Ierissou and Agion Oros. Fr. Peter is the founder and first editor of "Divine Ascent, A Journal of Orthodox Faith" (begun in 1995) and was the host of the podcast, "Postcards from Greece." He is the author of *The Missionary Origins of Modern Ecumenism: Milestones Leading up to 1920*, as well as *The Ecclesiological Renovation of the Second Vatican Council: An Orthodox Examination of Rome's Ecumenical Theology Regarding Baptism and the Church*, which was released in November of 2015. Fr. Peter is also the translator of several books, including the *Life of Elder Paisios* (co-translator) and the Epistles of Elder Paisios, *The Truth of our Faith* (vols. 1 & 2) by Elder Cleopa, *Apostle to Zaire: The Life of Fr. Cosmas of Grigoriou*, as well as the best-selling children's book *From I-ville to You-ville*. From January of 2017 until May of 2018, Fr. Peter was the instructor of Old and New Testament at Holy Trinity Orthodox Seminary in Jordanville, New York, and continues now as a Lecturer of Ecclesiology in the Certificate of Theological Studies

Program. From May of 2018 until December of 2019 he was the Headmaster of Three Hierarchs Academy in Florence, Arizona. Fr. Peter is the founder and current head of Uncut Mountain Press (founded in 2000), and founder of the Orthodox Ethos.

Deacon Ananias Sorem, Ph.D., is an Orthodox apologist and Professor of Philosophy at Fullerton College and Carroll College. He has taught philosophy at other universities, including University College Dublin, Azusa Pacific University, and Cal State Fullerton. He has a B.A. in Liberal Arts from Thomas Aquinas College (double major: philosophy and theology; double minor: math and science), together with an M.A. (Honors) and Ph.D. in Philosophy (specializing in epistemology, philosophy of science, and philosophy of mind) from University College Dublin. Deacon Ananias also attended the Diaconal Vocations Program at St. Vladimir's Orthodox Theological Seminary in Crestwood, New York. His current academic work focuses on philosophical theology, epistemology, and the philosophy of science. Deacon Ananias is the author of several articles and peer-reviewed papers, including: "Searle, Materialism, and the Mind-Body Problem," "Gnostic Scientism and Technocratic Totalitarianism," "An Orthodox Approach to the Dangers of Modernity and Technology," and "An Orthodox Theory of Knowledge: The Epistemological and Apologetic Methods of the Church Fathers." He is also the founder and editor-in-chief of the Orthodox website and online ministry, Patristic Faith. Deacon served at St. Mary's Romanian Orthodox Church in Anaheim, California, for four years before moving to Montana, where he resides with his wife Katherine. He serves at Holy Trinity Serbian Orthodox Church in Butte, Montana.

Presbytera Katherine Baker was born into a devout Roman Catholic family and spent much of her teens and early twenties as a Catholic catechist. She received a B.A. in English from Christendom College in Virginia and converted to the Orthodox faith in 2001, following a summer study abroad program in Juneau, Alaska. Her fiancé, Matthew Baker, was also studying his way toward the faith and the two converted together and married a few months later. They lived frugally and homeschooled their growing family while he attended Orthodox seminary. With her enthusiastic support, Matthew was finally ordained in the Greek Archdiocese in 2014 while pursuing his Ph.D. in theology. By then Presbytera Katherine had given birth to six children—five boys and one girl—and strove to make a home conducive to study and prayer, while stretching the tight finances. Father Matthew was assigned to his first parish but was killed only six weeks later in an automobile accident, when her oldest child was twelve and her youngest was two. Fordham University awarded Father Mathews the Ph.D. degree posthumously in 2015. Several of his essays and books were published. The latest, *Faith Seeking Understanding: The Theological Witness of Father Matthew Baker*, is available through St Vladimir Seminary Press. Presbytera Katherine and her children have been blessed by the generosity of the Church and have found solace in their faith. Her essays are available at IntellectualTakeout. org, Mercatornet.com, and Medium.com. A previous version of her essay in this volume, "A Pandemic Observed," has been widely shared and translated into several languages.

Irene Polidoulis, MD, CCFP, FCFP, was born in Athens Greece, and came to Canada at the age of four. She graduated from the *Faculty of Medicine* (MD) at the *University of Toronto* in 1984, followed by the completion of a two-year Family Medicine Residency Program at the *University of Saskatchewan* and a *Canadian Certificate in Family Practice* (CCFP) in 1986. She then returned to Toronto, where she began practising Family Medicine and raising a family. In 2002 she became a *Fellow of the College of Family Physicians of Canada* (FCFP). In 2008 she was promoted to Assistant Professor in the *Department of Family and Community Medicine* (DFCM) at the University of Toronto. During her medical education and career, Dr. Polidoulis has received several scholarships, nominations, and awards, including the CFPC Ontario Chapter *Award of Excellence* in 2013, the DFCM *Excellence in Creative Professional Activity* Award in 2014, and the Osteoporosis Canada (OC) Backbone Award in 2015 for her work on OC's Scientific Advisory Council and the Canadian Osteoporosis Patient Network. In addition, she has been involved in a variety of community activities, presentations, research articles, patient education materials and clinical tools involving knowledge translation. Born and raised Orthodox, Dr. Polidoulis taught Sunday School at her parish for many years, after graduating from the program herself. She strives to be a strong advocate for truth and considers her greatest blessings to be her Orthodox Faith and her loving and supportive husband and family. The opinions expressed by her in this book are her own, and do not represent the opinions of her medical department or faculty.

UNCUT MOUNTAIN PRESS TITLES

Books by Archpriest Peter Heers

Fr. Peter Heers, *The Ecclesiological Renovation of Vatican II: An Orthodox Examination of Rome's Ecumenical Theology Regarding Baptism and the Church*, 2015

Fr. Peter Heers, *The Missionary Origins of Modern Ecumenism: Milestones Leading up to 1920*, 2007

Works of our Father among the Saints, Nikodemos the Hagiorite

Vol. 1: *Exomologetarion: A Manual of Confession*

Vol. 2: *Concerning Frequent Communion of the Immaculate Mysteries of Christ*

Vol. 3: *Confession of Faith*

More Available Titles

Elder Cleopa of Romania, *The Truth of our Faith, Vol. I: Discourses from Holy Scripture on the Tenants of Christian Orthodoxy*

Elder Cleopa of Romania, *The Truth of our Faith, Vol. II: Discourses from Holy Scripture on the Holy Mysteries*

Fr. John Romanides, *Patristic Theology: The University Lectures of Fr. John Romanides*

Archimandrite Ephraim Triandaphillopoulos, *Noetic Prayer as the Basis of Mission and the Struggle Against Heresy*

G.M. Davis, *Antichrist: The Fulfillment of Globalization - The Ancient Church and the End of History*

Robert Spencer, *The Church and the Pope*

Select Forthcoming Titles

St. Gregory Palamas, *Apodictic Treatise on the Procession of the Holy Spirit*

The Lives and Witness of 20th Century Athonite Fathers

Protopresbyter Anastasios Gotsopoulos, *On Common Prayer with the Heterodox, According to the Canons of the Church*

St. Hilarion Troitsky, *An Overview of the History of the Dogma Concerning the Church*

Elder George of Grigoriou, *Catholicism*

Nicholas Baldimtsis, *Life and Witness of St. Iakovos of Evia*

Met. Neophytos of Morphou, *Homilies of Metropolitan Neophytos: Experiences with Contemporary Saints*

Georgio Kassir, *Errors of the Latins*

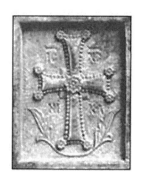

This 1st Edition of

LET NO ONE FEAR DEATH

having Fr. Alexander Webster and Fr. Peter Heers a:
editors, typeset in Baskerville and printed in this twc
thousandth and twenty second year of our Lord':
Holy Incarnation, is one of the many fine title:
available from Uncut Mountain Press, translators anc
publishers of Orthodox Christian theological anc
spiritual literature. Find the book you are looking for a

w w w . u n c u t m o u n t a i n p r e s s . c o m

Made in the USA
Columbia, SC
17 June 2022